Clinical Oncology: A Textbook for Students

Dr Anthony J. Neal, MRCP, FRCR
Clinical Research Fellow and Honorary
Senior Registrar in Clinical Oncology
The Institute of Cancer Research and
The Royal Marsden Hospital, Sutton,
Surrey, UK

and

Dr Peter J. Hoskin MD, MRCP, FRCR
Consultant in Clinical Oncology,
Mount Vernon Hospital, Northwood,
Middlesex, UK and Senior Lecturer in
Oncology, University College London
Medical School, UK

D1354296

Edward Arnold
A member of the Hodder Headline Group
LONDON   BOSTON   MELBOURNE   AUCKLAND

© 1994 Anthony J. Neal and Peter J. Hoskin

First published in Great Britain 1994

Distributed in the Americas by Little, Brown and Company
34 Beacon Street, Boston, MA 02108

British Library Cataloguing in Publication Data

Hoskin, Peter
   Clinical Oncology:Textbook for Students
   I. Title   II. Neal, Anthony J.
   616.992

   ISBN 0–340–59436–5

Typeset in 10/11pt Palatino by Anneset, Weston-super-Mare,
Avon. Printed and bound in Great Britain for Edward Arnold,
a division of Hodder Headline PLC, 338 Euston Road, London
NW1 3BH by St Edmundsbury Press Ltd, Bury St Edmunds,
Suffolk and Hartnolls Ltd, Bodmin, Cornwall.

Contents

Acknowledgements

We would like to express our gratitude to those of our colleagues who have provided clinical material for some of the figures, namely Dr D. Tait, Dr R. Thomas and Dr J. Yarnold, and to other sources including Isotopen-Technik (Dr Sauerwein Gmbh) and Philips Medical Systems.

Introduction

Of the 277 000 deaths registered in England and Wales in 1990, 76 000 were due to malignant disease (Fig. 1). Thus approximately 1 in 4 people will die from cancer in a given year, and of course many more will develop cancer but be successfully treated for it. The 10 most common cancers in men and women are outlined in Figure 2, and the mortality statistics for each cancer in Table 1. The management of such patients will therefore form a significant part of the daily practice of most doctors in clinical specialties.

This concise but detailed textbook has been written primarily for undergraduates in medicine to provide a readily available source of information on the epidemiology, aetiology, pathology, presentation, staging, management and prognosis for any chosen malignancy and to provide a foundation for their clinical training and practice. Recent advances and topical

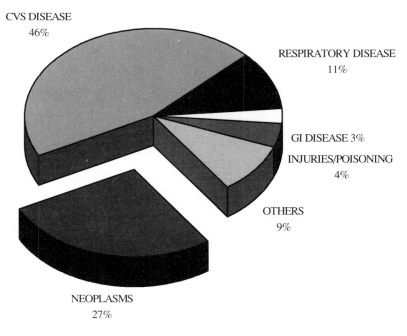

Fig. 1 Percentages for total number of deaths from all causes.

issues such as cancer screening and prevention are covered. There are also chapters dealing with the more general principles of patient management in the context of clinical oncology. Some basic prior knowledge of anatomy, physiology, medicine, surgery and radiology is assumed. Much of the content is also relevant to nurses working on oncology units and therapy radiographers who wish to acquire a core of basic knowledge in clinical oncology.

A. J. Neal and P. J. Hoskin
October 1993

Table 1   Mortality statistics for the most common cancers. (Adapted from The Cancer Research Campaign cancer factsheets).

Males

Site	No. of new cases p.a.[1]	No. of deaths[1]	5 year survival[2]
Lung	29 000	27 000	8%
Skin	16 000	300	97%
Prostate	12 000	9 000	43%
Bladder	8 000	4 000	62%
Colon	8 000	6 000	38%
Stomach	7 000	6 000	11%
Rectum	6 000	4 000	7%
Oesophagus	3 000	4 000	36%
Pancreas	3 000	3 000	4%

Females

Site	No. of new cases p.a.[1]	No. of deaths[1]	5 year survival[2]
Breast	27 000	15 000	62%
Skin	14 000	200	97%
Lung	13 000	12 000	7%
Colon	10 000	7 000	37%
Ovary	6 000	4 000	28%
Stomach	5 000	4 000	10%
Rectum	5 000	3 000	36%
Cervix	5 000	2 000	58%
Uterus	4 000	1 000	70%
Pancreas	3 000	3 000	4%

[1] UK figures rounded to the nearest 1 000
[2] England and Wales figures.

MALES:

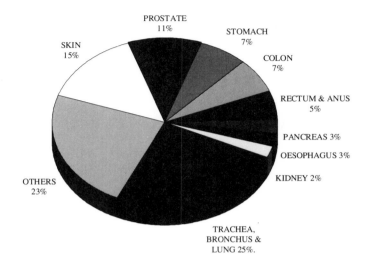

PROSTATE
11%

STOMACH
7%

SKIN
15%

COLON
7%

RECTUM & ANUS
5%

PANCREAS 3%

OESOPHAGUS 3%

OTHERS
23%

KIDNEY 2%

TRACHEA,
BRONCHUS &
LUNG 25%.

FEMALES:

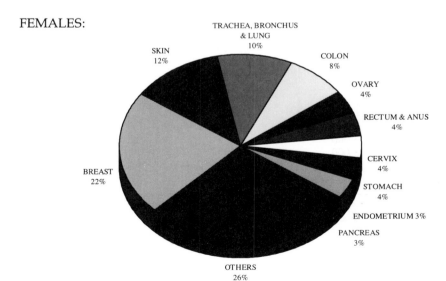

TRACHEA, BRONCHUS
& LUNG
10%

SKIN
12%

COLON
8%

OVARY
4%

RECTUM & ANUS
4%

BREAST
22%

CERVIX
4%

STOMACH
4%

ENDOMETRIUM 3%

PANCREAS
3%

OTHERS
26%

Fig. 2 The 10 most common cancers according to sex.

1

Pathogenesis of cancer

Pathogenesis is defined as 'the manner of development of a disease'. An understanding of the causes of a given cancer is an integral part of formulating strategies for successful treatment, screening and prevention. We owe much of our current understanding to epidemiologists who have discovered associations between different cancers and a number of genetic and environmental factors. In many cases, these lead directly to malignancy, e.g. smoking and lung cancer. The causative factors can be divided into genetic, chemical, physical and viral. It is becoming increasingly clear that changes in the host genome are the final common pathway in the process of carcinogenesis whatever the initial aetiology. However, in many patients with cancer it is still not possible to identify why that particular person developed cancer.

Genetic factors

The chromosomes contain the genetic material of the cell made up of deoxyribonucleic acid (DNA) which codes for proteins responsible for all the basic metabolic processes that enable the individual cells to survive, reproduce and express properties characteristic of their tissue of origin. Subtle changes in the genes comprising the chromosome may lead to a malignant tumour characterized by loss of the normal cellular mechanisms responsible for control of proliferation, cell differentiation, programmed cell death (apoptosis), cellular organization and cellular adhesion. The uncoupling of the usual balance between cell loss and multiplication leads to growth of the tumour (Fig. 1.1) and its subsequent invasion both locally and at distant sites.

The field of molecular biology has made great progress in understanding the cause of cancer at a number of sites. Much of this is due to the development of techniques for the isolation and identification of genetic material such as the polymerase chain reaction and gel electrophoresis. It is becoming apparent that most cancer patients have some form of genetic abnormality, the most common of which is a mutation of the p53 gene, the precise function of which is currently the subject of intense research.

The genetic aberrations associated with cancer can be classified as:

1. Activated oncogenes – these are genes which when expressed code for a protein which in some way is related to the proliferative cycle

of cells or cell differentiation. These products may be growth factors, growth factor receptors on the cell surface or the chemicals that transmit the receptor signals from the cytoplasm to the nucleus. Their overexpression or amplification leads to uncoupling of the usual cell loss/gain equilibrium in favour of cell multiplication, resulting in an increase in cell numbers and ultimately a palpable tumour. These oncogenes are well preserved throughout the evolutionary scale, remaining very similar right down to primitive organisms such as yeasts. They are activated during the intense cell proliferation and differentiation of embryogenesis but in the mature cells are suppressed by regulating genes further along the chromosome. DNA strand breaks (e.g. due to ionizing radiation or chemical carcinogens) with aberrant repair or translocations of genetic material may lead to loss of oncogene regulation which in turn leads to its activation. Similarly, if a point mutation leads to gene loss in the region of the regulator, again the oncogene may be inappropriately activated. Examples of oncogenes include ras, myc, neu, src and sis, each of which is singly or collectively amplified or overexpressed in specific types of cancer. The best characterized example is that

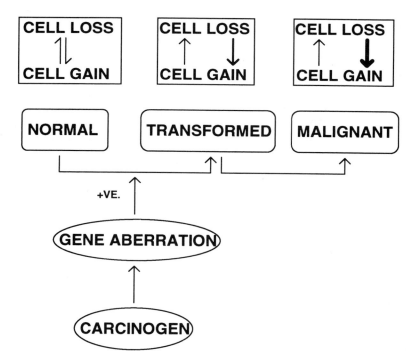

Fig. 1.1   Schematic representation of the development of a tumour within a tissue. A carcinogen (e.g. virus, chemical, physical phenomenon) induces an abnormality in the DNA sequence which leads to a gene aberation. This in turn leads to an uncoupling of the cell loss/gain equillibrium in favour of cell multiplication.

of the Philadelphia chromosome of chronic lymphatic leukaemia which is confined to the malignant clone and can be identified in 95 per cent of patients with the disease. There is a translocation of part of chromosome 9 to chromosome 22, placing the abl oncogene from chromosome 9 adjacent to the breakpoint cluster region (bcr) on chromosome 22. The fusion abl–bcr gene product leads to the leukaemic transformation by increasing lymphocyte proliferation.

2. Tumour suppressor genes – each cell has one of a pair of tumour suppressor genes on each homologous chromosome, and both must be lost for the cancer to develop. This means that individuals from a 'cancer family' with only a single gene inherited have a normal phenotype, act as a carrier, but will develop cancer if the second gene is lost due to a mutation or other form of genetic miscoding. Normal individuals must lose both genes spontaneously for a sporadic cancer to develop. This phenomenon accounts for cancer families where members are at risk from a given cancer (e.g. breast) or several cancers (e.g. breast, ovary, colon) but also explains the development of such cancers in 'normal' families. Examples include the retinoblastoma gene which is located on chromosome 13, Wilm's tumours and chromosome 11, and the familial polyposis coli gene which is located on chromosome 5.

Examples of inherited diseases associated with the development of cancer include:

1. Autosomal dominant:

   - Familial polyposis coli (adenoma/carcinoma of the colon/rectum).
   - Gardener's syndrome (adenoma/carcinoma of the colon/rectum).
   - Multiple endocrine adenomatosis types 1 and 2 (see Chapter 14).
   - Von Recklinghausen's disease (neurofibromas, schwannoma, phaeochromocytoma).
   - Palmar/plantar tylosis (carcinoma of the oesophagus).
   - Gorlin's syndrome (basal cell carcinoma of skin, medulloblastoma).
   - Von Hippel-Lindau disease (cerebellar haemangioblastoma, hypernephroma).

2. Autosomal recessive:

   - Albinism (melanoma, basal cell and squamous cell carcinomas of the skin).
   - Xeroderma pigmentosum (melanoma, squamous and basal cell carcinomas of the skin).
   - Ataxia telangiectasia (acute leukaemia).
   - Fanconi anaemia (acute leukaemia).
   - Wiscott–Aldrich syndrome (acute leukaemia).
   - Bloom's syndrome (acute leukaemia).

3. Chromosomal disorders:

   - Down's syndrome – trisomy 21 (acute leukaemia).
   - Turner's syndrome – XO (dysgerminoma).

Chemical factors

Cigarette smoking

Polycyclic aromatic hydrocarbons in the tar (e.g. benzpyrene) rather than the nicotine are carcinogenic. Smoking is strongly associated with carcinomas of the lung (squamous and small cell variants), oral cavity, larynx and bladder.

Asbestos

A history of asbestos is usually elicited from dockers, plumbers, builders and engineers and is associated with carcinomas of the lung, and mesotheliomas of the pleura and peritoneum. The blue variant is particularly carcinogenic.

Products of the rubber and aniline dye industry

Both beta naphthylamine and azo dyes are carcinogenic. These substances and their products are excreted in the urine, and cause cancers of the renal pelves, ureters and bladder.

Wood dust

Inhalation of hardwood dusts has been associated with adenocarcinoma of the nasal sinuses, first described in workers in the furniture factories of High Wycombe.

Soot

During the days of chimney sweeps, there was an increased risk of carcinoma of the scrotum due to trapping of soot in the rugosity of the scrotal skin and poor personal hygiene.

Tar/bitumen

As with cigarette smoke, polycyclic aromatic hydrocarbons may lead to cancer of exposed skin.

Mineral oils

An increased risk of skin cancer was noted in mule spinners due to exposure to lubricating oils.

Chromates, nickel

These are associated with the development of lung cancer.

Arsenic

Its use as a 'tonic' during the early 20th century led to multiple basal and squamous cell carcinomas of the skin. It has also been associated with lung cancer.

Aflatoxin

This is a product of the fungus *Aspergillus fumigatus*, which is a contaminant of poorly stored cereals and nuts, and causes hepatocellular carcinoma.

Nitrosamines

These are products of the action of intestinal bacteria on nitrogenous compounds in ingested food and have been implicated in stomach cancer.

Vinyl chloride monomer

Industrial exposure has led to angiosarcomas of the liver.

Alkylating chemotherapy agents

The addition of alkyl groups to the DNA double helix drastically changes its configuration and leads to difficulty when the cell undergoes mitosis or meiosis, ultimately leading to loss and distortion of the genome. Prior use of these agents in the chemotherapy of lymphoma has led to an increased risk of AML in long-term survivors.

Physical factors

Physical factors may lead to direct damage of the genome comprising DNA strand breaks or point mutations, both of which may lead to an aberration either of the gene sequence or of the genes themselves. This is a phenomenon of everyday life and the changes are either repaired by cellular protection mechanisms or are so severe that the cell perishes and does not multiply. However, if the effects are such that these mechanisms for repair are overloaded, the cell may divide and the genetic error expresses itself, possibly leading to a cell with a malignant phenotype. As the skin and mucosal surfaces are exposed to the external environment, it is these that are most prone to physical carcinogenic influences.

Solar radiation

Excessive ultraviolet exposure in normal individuals or minimal amounts in susceptible individuals (e.g. albinos, xeroderma pigmentosum) may lead to melanoma, basal cell carcinoma and squamous carcinoma.

Ionizing radiation

Several categories of exposure can be identified and implicated in carcinogenesis:

1. Excessive background radiation – radon gas is colourless and odour-less, being a daughter product from the radioactive decay of uranium in the Earth's crust, particularly in granite-rich areas. It seeps into homes, and reaches its highest level during winter when ventilation of dwellings is at its minimum. When inhaled, solid α particle-emitting daughter products may be deposited on the bronchial epithelium leading eventually to lung cancer. Uranium miners are at particular risk, and many have died of lung cancer in Czechoslovakia and Germany. Japanese atomic bomb survivors have an increased incidence of a number of solid tumours, particularly of the breast and radioiodine exposure from atomic bomb test fallout has caused thyroid cancer. Radium ingested by watch dial painters has led to bone sarcomas due to concentration of the element in the skeleton.
2. Excessive diagnostic radiology exposure – there was an increased risk of carcinoma of the breast in a cohort of women who had many chest fluoroscopies to monitor iatrogenic pneumothoraces. The use of thoratrast (containing thorium which has similar properties to radium) as a contrast agent led to tumours of the hepatobiliary tract and nasal sinuses.
3. Therapeutic radiation – breast irradiation for postpartum mastitis causes breast cancer and there is an increased incidence of papillary carcinoma of the thyroid after thyroid irradiation. Soft tissue sarcomas may arise at the edge of a previously irradiated area and skin carcino-mas may arise in previously irradiated skin.

Heat

Carcinomas of the skin have been described in chronic burn scars and the skin of Indians who wear heating lamps against their skin for warmth. Claypipe smokers are at risk of carcinoma of the lip.

Chronic trauma/inflammation

Carcinomas may arise at sites of chronic skin/mucosal damage (e.g. tongue adjacent to sharp teeth or a syphilitic lesion), at the site of a sinus from chronic osteomyelitis or inflammatory bowel disease, chronic venous (Marjolin's) ulcer on the lower limb, or colonic carcinoma after chronic ulcerative colitis. Calculi and the associated infection may predispose to carcinomas of the urinary and hepatobiliary tracts.

Viral factors

Viruses reproduce by integrating their own genes with those of the infected host, and in doing so the gene sequence of host chromosomes is adjusted. This may in turn lead to deregulation of genes which code for proteins involved in the proliferation of cells, which in turn leads to tumour development. Geographical regions where the virus is endemic will also be the sites of case clustering of the tumour. Evidence that a viral infection has led to a tumour includes:

1. Appropriate serological evidence of infection.
2. Visualization of viral particles in the tumour cells.
3. Identification of viral genome in the tumour DNA.

Hepatitis B

There is a high incidence of hepatoma in parts of Africa, where hepatitis B is endemic, and the tumour arises at a younger age than sporadic cases in the UK.

Epstein–Barr virus (EBV)

There is very strong evidence that this is the causative agent of nasopharyngeal carcinoma in Southeast Asia where it is the most common form of malignant disease.

Human papilloma virus (HPV)

HPV types 16 and 18 are responsible for warts in humans and are associated with carcinomas of the cervix and anal canal.

Human T-cell lymphotropic virus type 1 (HTLV-1)

This is a retrovirus related to the human immunodeficiency virus (HIV). It causes adult T-cell lymphoma leukaemia in the endemic regions of Japan and the Caribbean where more than 95 per cent of cases have positive viral serology.

Immune factors

There is evidence that the body's immunosurveillence system mediated by T-cells is capable of mounting an immune response to tumour cells. This is manifested as a lymphocytic infiltrate in tumours such as seminoma and melanoma, which correlates with a favourable prognosis, the phenomenon of spontaneous regression in hypernephroma and melanoma, and the objective responses seen when the T-cell population is boosted by cytokines such as interleukin 2 and interferon. There is evidence that immunosuppression leads to development of some forms of cancer, some of which are mediated by viruses.

Acquired immune deficiency syndrome (AIDS)

Up to 40 per cent of patients will ultimately develop some form of malignant disease, particularly Kaposi's sarcoma and non-Hodgkin's lymphoma.

Drug-induced myelosuppression

Transplant recipients receiving steroids and azothioprine or cyclosporin have an increased incidence of Kaposi's sarcoma, non-Hodgkin's lymphoma and skin cancer.

Endocrine factors

Many cells have receptors for hormones on their surface, within their cytoplasm and nucleus. Overstimulation of these receptors by endogenous or exogenous hormones may lead to excessive cell proliferation, usually resulting in an adenomatous change but sometimes malignancy.

Oestrogens

Excessive endogenous steroids (e.g. from a granulosa cell tumour of the ovary) or long-term exogenous oestrogens (e.g. high dose oestrogen-only oral contraceptive or hormone replacement therapy) may predispose to hyperplasia of the endometrium which may progress to a well-differentiated adenocarcinoma.

Trophic hormones

Excess physiological secretion of hormones may lead to hyperplasia, adenomatous change and eventually malignant transformation. For example, chronic severe iodine deficiency leads to a rise in TSH, leading to goitre and in some cases follicular carcinoma.

Understanding the cause of cancer – contribution to patient care

Identification of the aetiological agents for cancers is vital for identifying individuals at high risk. Avoiding exposure of employees to industrial carcinogens either by the issue of protective clothing or restricted access is a vital part of health and safety practice to prevent cancers. Similarly, screening of asymptomatic individuals may be indicated, e.g. regular urine cytology in rubber workers at risk of bladder cancer. Identification of cancer patients in whom industrial exposure to a carcinogen is implicated will entitle the patient to industrial injuries compensation. Understanding the cause of cancer also forms the backbone of more general health education programmes aimed at reducing tobacco consumption and exposure to excessive ultraviolet irradiation.

Molecular biology has already given us a particularly valuable insight into the mechanisms of carcinogenesis. Specific applications include:

1. Risk factor determination, prevention and genetic counselling – greater appreciation of the genetic origins of cancer will lead to the possibility of being able to assign a score to a patient's genome which will give some measure of their risk of developing cancer. This will make it possible to give individual counselling to a patient with regard to lifestyle adjustments that can be expected to lower that risk. In high risk families, it is already possible to counsel prospective parents as to the risk of their children acquiring an unduly high risk of cancer.
2. Screening – members of high risk families may be screened for the appropriate tumour suppressor genes. If both are found to be deleted, then appropriate prophylactic measures and/or close surveillance can be implemented.
3. Therapy – the ultimate goal of such research must be to give a greater understanding of cancer and ultimately facilitate cancer cure. An understanding of oncogene products will permit therapies to be precisely targeted at the molecular level to the cell receptor or its chemical messengers en route to the nucleus. The identification of precise genetic abnormalities may in turn enable cell biologists to insert the appropriate genetic code into the genome and thereby reverse the cellular processes of malignancy.

2

Principles of cancer diagnosis and staging

Diagnosis and staging are integral steps in the management of cancer patients.

The importance of obtaining a tissue diagnosis

Cancer treatment usually involves major procedures with significant toxicity and the diagnosis of cancer has profound psychological, social and physical consequences for the patient. It is therefore mandatory to be certain of the diagnosis before informing the patient or starting therapy. This may entail a simple biopsy or a more invasive procedure such as a laparotomy or craniotomy. As a rule of thumb, the least invasive means of obtaining tissue should be employed. However, occasionally, several attempts at obtaining tissue from an ill-defined and poorly accessible tumour prove unsuccessful or the patient may be unfit to undergo an essential procedure by virtue of age or general condition. Under these circumstances, clinical judgement and common sense must prevail. Clearly it would be inappropriate to investigate exhaustively an elderly and infirm person with an extensive asymptomatic brain tumour or widespread metastatic disease if no treatment or change in management would be considered. Specific methods of obtaining tumour tissue include the following.

Cytology of body fluids

A small specimen of body fluid (e.g. sputum, ascitic fluid, pleural fluid, urine, cerebrospinal fluid) may be spun down and the cells in it stained and examined under the microscope within minutes of its collection. An experienced cytologist can then give an immediate and accurate diagnosis. The false positive rate is low although false negatives occur due to errors in interpretation or sampling. This analysis has the advantage that the specimen can often be collected as an outpatient with minimal discomfort and gives a result quickly so that treatment can start as soon as possible.

Cytology of tissue scrapings

Superficial cells are removed from a body surface (e.g. skin, vagina, cervix, bronchial mucosa, oesophageal mucosa) by scraping or brushing, before being stained and examined under the microscope. The advantages and limitations are the same as for fluid cytology.

Fine needle aspiration (FNA)

This entails the passage of a fine gauge hypodermic needle into a suspected tumour under local anaesthetic. Ultrasound or CT guidance may be necessary for deep-seated tumours that cannot be palpated such as those at the lung apex or retroperitoneum. Cells are aspirated, smeared onto a microscope slide and sent to a cytologist. This method is particularly useful for discriminating between reactive and malignant lymphadenopathy and for assessing breast lumps.

Needle biopsy

This is more invasive than FNA. A core of tissue is taken with a biopsy needle (e.g. Trucut) under local anaesthetic and the specimen is sectioned after fixing and mounting in wax, which means that the result will not be available for several days after collection. The larger specimen makes a false negative result less likely.

Incision biopsy

A small ellipse of tissue is taken from the edge of the tumour using a small scalpel under local anaesthetic. A punch biopsy instrument can be used instead of a scalpel to obtain a core of tissue, but this is more traumatic.

Excision biopsy

The tumour is excised *in toto* with a narrow margin of normal tissue. Unlike the other investigations, this has the advantage of removing the lesion which may be curative for benign tumours and certain skin malignances if the microscopic margins are clear. It can, however, make further management difficult if the original boundaries of the tumour are not apparent after excision.

Principles of cancer staging

Once the diagnosis has been confirmed, the stage of the cancer which defines the size and extent of the tumour must be ascertained. Staging has several purposes:

1. It indicates the most appropriate treatment – staging entails a detailed assessment as to the local extent of the tumour and whether there is evidence of spread elsewhere, e.g. regional lymphatics, distant

metastases. This will in turn help the referring specialist and oncologist to decide on what is the most appropriate therapy. For example, a patient with distant metastases is unlikely to be a candidate for aggressive surgery to remove the primary tumour but may be a candidate for systemic treatment such as chemotherapy. Alternatively, the detection of lymph node metastases alone may indicate to the surgeon that excision of the primary tumour should be combined with a lymph node dissection and/or systemic adjuvant therapy. Detailed surgical staging is also valuable to the radiotherapist in deciding the volume of tissue to be irradiated.

2. It permits assessment of the response to treatment – a thorough assessment of the tumour dimensions prior to therapy will permit a critical evaluation of the response to treatment at a later date. Accurate measurements in two planes perpendicular to each other can be used as a crude measure of tumour size before, during and after therapy.

3. It provides a guide to the likely prognosis – in most cancers, the ultimate outcome and therefore life expectancy is related to the stage. Patients with metastatic disease at presentation will clearly fare worse than patients with disease localized to the site of origin. The only tumours that are potentially curable when distant metastases are present are seminoma, teratoma, choriocarcinoma, lymphoma and leukaemia.

4. It standardizes the recording of clinical data – the vast body of retrospectively gathered clinical data that has guided generations of clinicians relies on accurate recording of stage to allow clinicians to assess its meaning and validity, and also enables true comparisons between similar patients in trials of new treatments.

Staging may be clinical, based on the clinician's history and examination, non-clinical, comprising blood tests and radiological studies, and pathological, based on the surgical specimen.

History

A thorough and systematic history can reveal symptoms that may suggest the need for specific staging investigations or a certain disease stage. For example, systemic symptoms such as weight loss, anorexia, malaise and fever raise the suspicion of metastatic disease. Specific symptoms at a site away from the primary tumour may also be suspicious of distant metastases, e.g. skeletal pain, early morning headache, haemoptysis, hepatic pain.

Examination

A full physical examination should be performed in all cases. The primary tumour's size, shape, position and mobility should be recorded, preferably with a diagram. The regional lymph nodes should be carefully palpated – involved nodes are enlarged, usually non-tender, hard and may be fixed to each other, the overlying skin or underlying tissues. The sclerae should be examined for jaundice and the abdomen palpated for hepatomegaly in which the liver is typically hard and knobbly. The chest is examined for signs of collapse, consolidation or effusion. The skin should be surveyed for any abnormal appearances which may be biopsied if suspicious. A detailed neurological examination should be performed to exclude focal or global neurological deficit, and the fundi examined to exclude papilloedema. Tenderness over sites of bone pain is suspicious and should be followed by appropriate radiographs.

Investigations

A knowledge of the patterns of spread of tumours will aid the selection of staging investigations. All patients should have a full blood count, liver function tests, calcium and alkaline phosphatase. The interpretation of deranged values is outlined in Table 2.1. An ESR is useful in lymphoma and myeloma. A chest X-ray should be performed in all cases to exclude obvious pulmonary metastases, with equivocal cases proceeding to a CT scan of the thorax. In the case of bone/soft tissue sarcomas, a CT scan of the thorax is justified at the outset as this will be more sensitive and spare the patient major surgery.

Other imaging may be indicated

1. Plain radiographs of the skeleton – films should be taken of the site of any unexplained bone pain, particularly if affecting a weight-bearing bone as these are prone to pathological fracture which can be prevented if the metastasis is detected early. A skeletal survey comprising views of the skull, thoracic spine, lumbar spine and pelvis is indicated in suspected myeloma but for other cancers a bone scan is more appropriate when there are widespread skeletal symptoms.
2. Liver ultrasound – this should be performed in all gastrointestinal malignancies as these metastasize to the liver via the portal circulation. It is sensitive, specific, non-invasive and more easily available than CT.
3. Isotope bone scan – this is indicated in tumours which frequently metastasize to the skeleton when potentially curative local therapy is

Table 2.1 Interpretation of abnormal screening blood tests

Test result	Interpretation
Normochromic normocytic anaemia	Suggests possibility of advanced cancer
Leucoerythroblastic anaemia	Suggests heavy bone marrow infiltration
Elevated alkaline phosphatase with normal gammaglutamyltransferase ± elevated calcium	Suggests possible bone metastases
Elevated alkaline phosphatase + gamma-glutamyltransferase ± bilirubin	Suggests possible liver metastases

being considered, e.g. carcinoma of the prostate, carcinoma of the breast, carcinoma of the lung. A metastasis is usually associated with an osteoblastic response in the surrounding bone which in turn leads to increased uptake of isotope and therefore a hot spot. Equivocal areas should be corroborated by plain radiographs.

4. Computed tomography (CT) – a CT scan of the thorax, abdomen and pelvis is indicated for potentially curable tumours with a propensity for widespread multiple metastases and is performed in all cases, e.g. lymphoma, germ cell tumours of the testis. A CT scan of the chest is valuable for excluding pulmonary metastases when the chest X-ray appearances are equivocal. A CT scan of the pelvis is valuable in tumours of the urogenital tract to delineate the extent of the primary and exclude enlarged lymph nodes. Abnormal lymph nodes on CT are defined as > 1 cm in diameter, although CT cannot detect abnormal lymph node architecture and therefore cannot distinguish between benign and malignant enlargement.

5. Magnetic resonance imaging (MRI) – this gives soft tissue contrast superior to that of CT and superb anatomical definition in transverse, sagittal and coronal views (Fig. 2.1). It is particularly useful in the central nervous system for defining the brain and spinal cord (where it is replacing myelography) and is also the investigation of choice in the delineation of the local extent of soft tissue sarcomas.

6. Lymphangiography – this entails the injection of a blue dye into the first web space of the foot which is taken up by lymphatics, permitting visualization and cannulation of a small lymph vessel and injection of radiographic contrast. Although largely superseded by CT, it does outline the architecture of pelvic and lower para-aortic nodes and identifies nodes of normal size with metastatic deposits. It also opacifies the nodes for many months allowing monitoring of disease status by serial plain radiographs.

Other specialized investigations include:

1. Bone marrow aspirate and trephine – lymphoma, small cell lung cancer, Ewing's sarcoma.
2. Serum acid phosphatase or prostatic specific antigen in prostate cancer.
3. Serum α foetoprotein (AFP) and β human chorionic gonadotrophin (HCG) in teratomas.
4. Calcitonin in medullary carcinoma of the thyroid.
5. 24 hour urinary vanilylmandelic acid (VMA) in phaeochromocytoma.
6. 24 hour 5-hydroxyindoleacetic acid (5HIAA) in carcinoid tumours.
7. Urinary Bence–Jones protein, serum paraprotein and immunoglobulin electrophoresis in myeloma.

Tumour markers in the serum are useful in many aspects of cancer management, and testis tumours provide a number of examples (Table 2.2).

(a)   (b)

(c)

Fig. 2.1 A MRI scan of the brain showing (a) transverse, (b) sagittal and (c) coronal (c) images. The scan shows a tumour arising from the pineal region.

Table 2.2 Role of serum tumour markers in the management of patients with testis tumours

Role	Example
Diagnosis	Elevation of AFP suggests teratomatous elements
Staging	Failure of AFP/HCG to return to normal after orchidectomy suggests residual disease elsewhere
Assessment of prognosis	Very high levels of AFP/HCG are associated with a poor prognosis
Indicator of response to treatment	Failure of AFP/HCG to fall with chemotherapy suggests resistant disease
Early detection of relapse	Sudden elevation of AFP/HCG while in clinical remission suggests subclinical relapse

The TNM staging system

The origins of this staging system go back to Pierre Denoix in the 1940s. Since then it has evolved into a comprehensive system covering all types and stages of cancer. It is accepted and contributed to by the most eminent cancer research groups such as the World Health Organization, International Union Against Cancer and International Society of Paediatric Oncology. A formalized, universally applied staging scheme has several advantages. First, it aids the clinician in his or her appreciation of the extent of the cancer and gives a meaningful guide to likely prognosis. Secondly, it gives a consistency in the reporting of clinical trials and facilitates an exchange of meaningful information between clinicians without ambiguity, even if they do not speak the same language. The system describes the anatomical extent of the disease by using three components:

1. 'T' for the primary tumour.
2. 'N' for regional lymph nodes.
3. 'M' for distant metastases.

Each of these is assigned a number corresponding to the extent of local and distant spread and are characteristic of a particular tumour. Other categories include:

Tis – Carcinoma *in situ*.
T0 – No evidence of primary.
Tx – Primary cannot be assessed.
Nx – Nodes cannot be assessed.
Mx – Metastases cannot be assessed.
G1 – Well differentiated.

G2 – Moderately differentiated.
G3 – Poorly differentiated.
G4 – Undifferentiated.
'pT/N/M' – Pathological staging.

The reader is referred to the site specific chapters for more detailed staging descriptions.

Use of pathological information

The pathologist plays a vital role in tumour diagnosis. The information on a pathology report is an integral part of the decision-making process for the clinician. Essential details include:

- Tumour size and macroscopic appearances.
- Tissue of origin.
- Benign v. malignant.
- If malignant, primary v. secondary.
- Degree of tumour differentiation.
- Degree of locoregional invasion (blood vessels, lymphatic vessels, nerve fibres, organ capsule, lymph nodes).
- Degree of host immune response.
- Whether the surgeon has completely excised the tumour with an adequate margin of normal tissue.

Much of this information is of prognostic value and may assist in determining the optimal treatment of the patient. The recent advances in immunocytochemistry have allowed pathologists to identify the tissue of origin in very poorly differentiated tumours (see Chapter 21) which has improved the management of this small group of patients. As with the radiologist, it is not only courteous but essential that as much relevant clinical information as possible is put onto any form submitted to the pathologist.

3

Decision making

The following chapters describe clear treatment policies for different types of malignant disease. These policies are based upon a knowledge of the natural history of the disease and, as detailed in the previous chapter, details of its extent – the clinical or pathological stage of the tumour.

However, the practice of clinical oncology demands more than simple application of these instructions in an uncritical fashion. The individualization of treatment for any given patient will be influenced by sociological, economic and psychological factors as well as oncological principles.

Three levels of decision making may be identified when formulating a treatment policy for an individual:

1. The decision to treat or not to treat.
2. Treatment intent, whether palliative or radical.
3. Specific aspects of treatment policy regarding local, systemic and supportive therapy.

To treat or not to treat

Not every patient in whom a diagnosis of cancer is made will benefit from active treatment of their disease. There is, for example, good evidence to show that active local treatment in the form of radiotherapy for inoperable carcinoma of the bronchus will have no impact whatsoever on the survival of a patient. It follows therefore that in asymptomatic patients diagnosed with this condition treatment will only be meddlesome and indeed may detract from that patient's quality of life by invoking side effects for no positive outcome. However, it is equally important that those patients who develop symptoms from a bronchial carcinoma are not denied treatment by operating a blanket policy of no treatment for these patients. The actual decision to treat a patient will be based not only on their clinical state but also on the availability of treatment facilities and the emotional response of the patient and their relatives. It is often very difficult for a patient to accept that having been told they have cancer no treatment is proposed beyond occasional visits to their doctor, even though the treatment may have no proven benefit.

A more comfortable scenario in which a no treatment decision may be taken is when the prognosis is so good and the risk of relapse so small that treatment for all patients will result in overtreatment with consequent side effects for the majority. An example of this situation is the management of stage 1 testicular teratoma following orchidectomy where the probability of relapse is around 20 per cent and the use of tumour markers and scans enables early diagnosis of relapse in a tumour which is readily cured on exposure to appropriate chemotherapy. This is a much easier scenario for the patient who will readily accept that they are almost certainly cured and require no further treatment other than close follow-up for a year or two.

Treatment should always have a positive benefit for the patient but treatment outcome is not entirely predictable. The decision to treat or not then becomes a matter of balancing the probability of improving a patient's condition, whether by symptom control with palliative treatment or by cure with radical treatment, against the toxicity and disturbance to lifestyle that treatment will entail. Thus it is possible to justify an intensive course of chemotherapy with major side effects when there is a high probability of cure but more difficult to do so in a patient with limited life expectancy in whom only minor symptom improvement can be anticipated.

Radical or palliative treatment

Radical treatment is that which is given with the intent of long-term control or cure for the patient. Palliative treatment is that which is given to improve the quality of life for a patient with no implied impact upon their survival.

While this may seem to be a clear distinction, in practice it may be difficult to define treatment aims in these terms. For example, a patient presenting with small cell lung cancer may be offered a course of radical treatment comprising intensive chemotherapy and perhaps also chest radiotherapy. However, it is recognized that while this treatment may prolong survival the likelihood of cure is less than 15 per cent. Thus the treatment intent, although radical, will result for most patients in only very limited benefit. Conversely a patient with breast cancer relapsing with a single site of painful bone metastases may receive a low palliative dose of radiation for pain relief only, yet live for several years.

In most cases, however, the decision of treatment intent if not outcome will be clear. Those patients who present with localized tumours accessible to local therapy and those with metastatic disease from chemosensitive tumours such as germ cell tumour or lymphoma will be offered radical treatment. Those who present with metastatic disease from other tumours and those who relapse after primary treatment will with few exceptions fall into the palliative group.

It should be noted that palliative treatment has the aim of improving a patient's well-being usually through treatment for specific local symptoms such as pain, obstruction or haemorrhage. It should follow therefore that patients who have cancer for which radical treatment is not appropriate and who have no symptoms do not require palliative treatment. The concept of prophylactic palliative treatment, in other words treatment to prevent symptoms emerging, is for most patients inappropriate and in the asymptomatic patient introduces treatment toxicity with little likelihood of benefit. There may be occasional exceptions to this concept, for example the prophylactic fixation of a bone with extensive osteolytic disease and impending pathological fracture. As always the probability of treatment benefit must be weighed against the natural history of the condition and probability of disease-related and treatment-related symptoms.

Local, regional or systemic treatment

As a general principle, a primary malignant tumour will require ablation with local treatment which may be surgical excision and/or radiation treatment. Similarly, metastatic disease requires systemic treatment which may be chemotherapy or hormone therapy.

Local treatment may involve simple excision of a tumour, removal of the entire organ or removal of the involved organ and regional tissues at risk of tumour involvement. In the past there have been advocates of extensive local surgery in the hope of improving cure, however such approaches are only rational where a tumour is known to develop locally and then spread in a predictable fashion. In practice most common tumours are thought to spread at an early stage in their evolution through blood and lymphatic dissemination of tumour cells. For this reason the use of radical regional surgery is usually inappropriate. This is well illustrated in the case of breast cancer where it is now clear that survival is largely independent of local treatment for a given stage of disease. Thus radical mastectomy is no better at curing breast cancer than simple removal of the lump from the breast.

Although local control of a tumour is an important goal most patients die from cancer because of metastatic disease. Where a cancer has been detected prior to the establishment of metastases then radical local treatment can result in cure. However, the natural history of many cancers is such that even relatively early tumours will already be associated with distant micrometastases. In these cases improvements in survival are likely to come only from the use of systemic treatment.

Adjuvant treatment

Adjuvant treatment is the prophylactic use of local or systemic treatment following primary treatment of a malignant tumour to prevent recurrence.

The most common form of adjuvant treatment given today is probably the use of post-operative radiotherapy following excision of a malignant tumour, for example irradiation of the breast following local excision of an early carcinoma. Such adjuvant treatment may add significantly to patient morbidity and it is important therefore to consider the relative merits of treatment or no treatment in these situations. For example, the risk of local relapse in the breast following simple excision with no radiotherapy is around 30–50 per cent depending upon tumour size. On this basis if all patients are treated following lumpectomy half may never have required treatment; the difficulty lies in predicting accurately those who will relapse. A further consideration is the fact that local relapse following lumpectomy may be treated successfully in many women and will still occur in 5–10 per cent even with radiotherapy. It has also been shown that adding radiotherapy to simple excision does not improve survival. The decision to offer a woman radiotherapy following excision of a malignant breast lump therefore has to balance the potential benefits with the likely side effects for each individual patient.

The use of adjuvant systemic therapy is also one in which decisions to offer a particular treatment may be questioned and where the acute morbidity is often considerable. There are in fact few sites of cancer where the use of adjuvant systemic therapy is of proven value. The area where there has been the greatest endeavour and the most reliable information is once again breast cancer. There is now little doubt that an overall survival benefit is achieved by offering women with early operable breast cancer some form of adjuvant systemic therapy. In post-menopausal women tamoxifen is recommended. This reduces the likelihood of dying from breast cancer by one-third and is a simple treatment involving the administration of a single tablet daily for a number of years with few if any associated side effects. Therefore the decision in this case is reasonably straightforward. In contrast there is a less reliable effect of tamoxifen in pre-menopausal women and at present chemotherapy is recommended. However, this treatment involves 6 months of intravenous chemotherapy with attendant side effects. Furthermore most evidence for its efficacy lies in those patients with positive axillary lymph nodes but even so the difference in survival at 10 years between women who receive chemotherapy and those who do not in prospective randomized trials is only 6 per cent. Therefore treatment decision for adjuvant chemotherapy in a pre-menopausal patient with negative lymph nodes in whom there may be only a small probability of advantage for the individual becomes more difficult.

It can be difficult to translate clinical trial and population-based data to the individual patient. Breast cancer is a common cancer and therefore even a very small treatment effect of, say, an improvement in survival of 5 per cent over 10 years will result in many thousands of women worldwide living for longer after breast cancer. However, for the individual woman the odds that she will benefit from adjuvant treatment in that setting are small and it is possible that she will undergo a toxic treatment with no effect on her ultimate survival.

It is also difficult for those around the patient, be they family, friends or physicians, to evaluate and balance the risks of having a toxic treatment against the risk of relapse, particularly when there can never be the certainty of cure. There is evidence to suggest that patients have a much lower threshold for accepting treatment, even where there is significant associated toxicity, than would the nurses or doctors who look after them.

Conclusion

Decision making in oncology is not as straightforward as a simple knowledge of the disease process may imply. Relating the large body of knowledge regarding disease outcome, treatment outcome and treatment-related morbidity to an individual patient can be difficult. The probability of benefit from any treatment may be interpreted differently by each patient so that while one might accept a 90 per cent probability of cure as very favourable, another will find a 10 per cent probability of relapse unacceptable. Treatment decisions rely on an accurate and realistic presentation of the facts but individual interpretations may come to very different conclusions from the same facts.

4

Principles of surgical oncology

The local treatment of malignant disease involves the use of surgery, radiotherapy or a combination of the two. Surgery is essentially a local treatment while radiotherapy offers locoregional treatment covering a wider area which is less constrained by anatomical boundaries and surgical technique.

Optimum initial management of the primary tumour and regional metastases is vital if later relapse is to be avoided, and close liaison between surgeon and clinical oncologist is required to enable the best use of each modality.

Management of the primary tumour

Surgery for a malignant tumour may have two or three components:

1. Tissue biopsy to establish the diagnosis.
2. Removal of malignant disease with a clear margin of normal tissue.
3. Repair, reconstruction and restoration of function. This may vary according to the extent of resection and anatomical site from simple primary wound closure to major reconstruction of bone and soft tissue with vascularized grafts and prostheses.

The type of surgery required will be determined by the type of tumour and the anatomical site, and may include any of the following:

1. Wide local excision of the tumour mass, e.g. local excision of a breast lump.
2. Removal of part of an organ and surrounding tissue, e.g. partial glossectomy and neck dissection for a carcinoma of the tongue.
3. Removal of an entire organ, e.g. laryngectomy, cystectomy or hysterectomy.

En bloc removal of the immediate lymphatic drainage areas is usually an integral part of any cancer surgery, e.g. hysterectomy for cervical cancer includes pelvic lymphadenectomy.

Radiotherapy will give equivalent local control rates to surgery for small tumours (< 5 cm) in many sites and has the potential advantage in certain sites of being able to preserve anatomical structure and function, e.g. in the treatment of cancer of the larynx where radical radiotherapy can result in tumour eradication with voice preservation in contrast to the surgical alternative which is total laryngectomy. However, against this must be balanced the need for close post-radiotherapy surveillance and that a significant proportion (around 20 per cent) of patients will still come to surgery. Furthermore surgery following radiotherapy may be technically more difficult and have a higher complication rate.

As with surgical management irradiation of a local tumour must include areas of potential spread. A common approach to enable high radiation doses to be concentrated at the site of the tumour mass is to use a shrinking field technique. This involves:

1.   Initial treatment of a wide area to cover all potential routes of microscopic spread together with the primary tumour and regional lymphatics.
2.   A boost to the primary tumour site alone with a margin of 1–2 cm.

Combined surgery and radiotherapy

This has two potential advantages and applications:

1.   To enable the extent of surgery to be limited by treating sites of microscopic disease immediately adjacent to the primary site with radiotherapy, e.g. the use of local excision and radiotherapy in place of mastectomy for breast cancer.
2.   For large tumours (> 5 cm) local control rates are in general better for combined therapy than either modality alone.

Combined treatment may involve the use of pre-operative or post-operative radiotherapy. The relative merits of each approach are shown in Table 4.1.

Table 4.1   Relative merits of pre- and post-operative radiotherapy

Pre-op RT	Post-op RT
Early radiotherapy	No delay to surgery
Enables pre-op preparation for planned surgery	True pathological staging may be masked by pre-op RT
Surgery may be easier if tumour shrinks pre-op	Pathology of surgical specimen may guide later RT
	Lower dose of RT needed for microscopic disease

There is no evidence that pre- or post-operative radiotherapy is more effective in ultimate tumour control.

Management of regional lymph nodes

The common epithelial tumours such as those of the lung, breast, head and neck region and pelvis metastasize through two routes: the lymph system and the blood circulation. Clinically involved lymph nodes and those at high risk of microscopic involvement require active treatment.

Surgery

Surgery is indicated for the immediate draining nodes around a primary tumour. Radical dissection of the involved node chain should be performed, e.g.:

- Axillary dissection for breast cancer.
- Radical neck dissection for head and neck sites.
- Inguinal node dissection for vulval, anal or penile cancers.

Radical excision of nodes is not indicated in the following situations:

- Lymphomas (Hodgkin's disease or non-Hodgkin's lymphoma) or leukaemias.
- Metastatic breast cancer involving the supraclavicular fossa or neck.
- Lymph nodes presenting as the sole manifestation of a malignancy from an unknown primary site.

Radiotherapy

Radiotherapy is indicated for surgically inoperable nodes and may succeed in rendering inoperable nodes operable.

Post-operative radiotherapy following surgical dissection is recommended for those patients with multiple node involvement and extension of tumour beyond the capsule of the gland.

Prophylactic radiotherapy to sites of potential microscopic disease is often given when treating a primary site, e.g. pelvic nodes for gynaecological malignancy, neck nodes for head and neck tumours.

Chemotherapy

Chemotherapy may be indicated for enlarged lymph nodes due to lymphoma, metastatic breast cancer or small cell lung cancer.

Palliative surgery

Even when cure is no longer a realistic aim surgery may have an important role in the palliation of local symptoms. Specific examples where surgery should be considered include the following.

Relief of obstructive symptoms

Palliative resection of a bowel tumour or a simple bypass procedure such as a gastrojejunostomy will avoid symptoms of intestinal obstruction.

Laser or cryotherapy resection of an obstructing tumour mass will restore the lumen of an obstructed bronchus or oesophagus.

Intubation of the oesophagus using a Celestin or Atkinson tube provides rapid and effective relief of dysphagia.

Nephrostomy or passage of pig-tail ureteric catheters will relieve obstructive hydronephrosis.

Biliary stents or choledochojejunostomy will relieve obstructive jaundice due to main bile duct obstruction as in carcinoma of the pancreas.

Ventriculoperitoneal shunting of hydrocephalus may result in dramatic improvement of headache and neurological deficits even though the underlying tumour may be incurable.

Control of haemorrhage

Diathermy at bronchoscopy or cystoscopy will control haemoptysis or haematuria.

Similarly bleeding tumours in the oesophagus, stomach or in the large bowel may be controlled using diathermy or laser coagulation at endoscopy.

Tumour fungation

Local resection even if not complete may be of value for a locally advanced tumour mass which is necrotic and breaking down. Toilet mastectomy for a progressive breast cancer is perhaps the most common example of this.

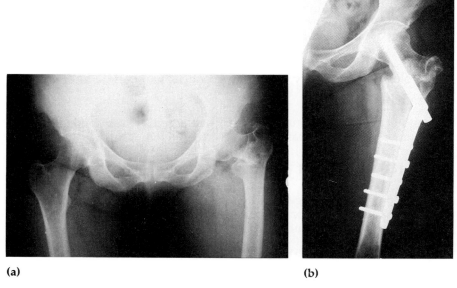

(a)   (b)

Fig. 4.1   Pathological fracture of the left neck of femur (a) before and (b) after internal fixation.

Fracture fixation

Pathological fracture of a weight-bearing bone is best dealt with by internal fixation followed by post-operative radiotherapy. In certain circumstances prophylactic fixation may also be indicated; specific indications for this include diffuse lytic bone disease in a weight-bearing area and destruction of more than 50 per cent per cent of the cortex by a lytic deposit. This is shown in Figure 4.1.

5

Principles of radiotherapy

Radiotherapy is the use of ionizing radiation to treat disease. Ionizing radiation may be delivered by X-ray beams, beams of ionizing particles, e.g. electrons, or by beta or gamma irradiation produced in the decay of radioactive isotopes.

Types of radiotherapy

External beam radiotherapy

External beam radiotherapy is the most common form of treatment in clinical use. A range of X-ray beams is available, varying according to their energy.

Superficial voltage

These X-ray beams are of energy 50–150 kV and are, as their name implies, suitable for the treatment of superficial lesion in the skin; their useful treatment energy penetrates to only 1 cm or so beneath the surface.

Orthovoltage machines

These produce X-rays of energy 200–300kV and penetrate to a depth of approximately 3 cm. These are therefore useful for treating structures such as ribs, scapula or sacrum but are not sufficiently powerful to reach deeper internal organs.

Megavoltage machines

These are either linear accelerators producing high energy X-ray beams of 4–20 MV or cobalt machines containing a source of cobalt-60 in their head which decays spontaneously to nickel-60 releasing gamma rays of 1.2 and 1.3 MV. Linear accelerators form the mainstay of modern clinical radiotherapy and are gradually superseding older cobalt machines as they come to the end of their working life. A modern linear accelerator is shown in Figure 5.1.

Electron beams are also produced by linear accelerators and have the advantage that as a particulate radiation beam they have a defined range in tissue with a sharp cut-off at the point where they deliver their energy.

This is of value where a tumour is superficial and overlying a radiosensitive structure such as the spinal cord.

Fig. 5.1 A modern linear accelerator (courtesy of Philips Medical Systems).

Brachytherapy

This is the use of radioactive sources placed either on or within a site of tumour. The great advantage of this form of treatment is the rapid fall off in dose at only a short distance from the source (obeying the inverse square law).

Mould treatment uses sources placed directly over a superficial tumour of the skin fixed in a plastic mounting (the mould).

Intracavitary treatment involves the placing of radioactive sources within a body cavity. Intrauterine tubes and vaginal sources in the treatment of gynaecological tumours are a common application of this technique.

Interstitial treatment involves the direct placing of radioactive needles or wire in the area of interest. This technique is used for cancer of the tongue, floor of mouth or breast.

The first isotope to be employed was radium. This is no longer used because it constitutes a major radiation hazard having a long half-life (1620 years) and decaying to a radioactive gas (radon). It has been superseded initially by cobalt sources and currently by caesium and iridium as the principal isotopes used for brachytherapy.

Direct handling

Direct handling of live sources is most commonly used today when iridium wire hairpins are inserted directly into the tumour area, typically the tongue or floor of mouth. Its major disadvantage is the exposure of staff and patients within the hospital to radiation from the time of insertion to the time of removal, which may be for several days. This means that careful monitoring is required and that there are limits to the time that individuals can spend in caring for the patient. It also means that members of the general public, including close relatives, are not permitted to be with the patient.

Manual afterloading

In this inactive source carriers are used initially to enable accurate siting of the treatment and so that the patient can be moved within the hospital from theatre or the X-ray department without active live sources. The active isotope is introduced manually once the patient has returned to their protected room and their post-operative recovery is complete.

Remote afterloading

In this, following placement of the source carriers, the radiation sources are introduced by remote control via pneumatic pipes or a cable connected to the source carriers within the patient. This system minimizes exposure to staff and in practice means that only the patient is exposed to radiation. It is also possible to interrupt the treatment so that the patient can receive attention without further exposing hospital personnel and with no time limits on their stay. A modern afterloading machine is shown in Figure 5.2.

Fig. 5.2 A modern brachytherapy afterloading machine (courtesy of Isotopen-Technik Dr Sauerwein Gmbh (Gammamed))

All such treatments require the patient to be isolated in a protected room with thickened or shielded walls, floors and ceilings. Treatments may last from 3 to 4 minutes for a high dose rate gynaecology treatment to several days for a radical interstitial treatment.

Internal isotope treatment

Internal isotope treatment involves the administration of a radioactive isotope systemically which is then concentrated within the body at certain sites. Specific examples of this form of treatment are the use of radioiodine (I-131) for thyroid cancer, phosphorus (P-32) for polycythaemia rubra vera and strontium (Sr-89) for bone metastases.

Other forms of radiation

There has been interest in forms of radiation other than X-rays or gamma rays for therapeutic use. These are either radiation which causes greater biological damage along each path track it traverses – high linear energy transfer (LET) radiation – or beams which have a highly focused deposition of radiation (Bragg peak).

Neutrons have been evaluated extensively in a number of centres across Europe and the US. Their advantages are that they have less dependence on oxygen for cell killing and cause more direct damage to the cellular DNA. While there is little doubt that they are more effective at achieving cell kill they are not selective for cancer cells and their use has been accompanied by unacceptably high levels of normal tissue damage and severe late side effects.

Protons are available in a few high energy cyclotron units around the world. Their advantage is the production of a highly localized, high energy peak in their beam which by manipulation of the beam energy and the use of absorbing materials can be focused to a defined position in a patient. Biologically they are similar in action to X-rays. They have been used particularly for tumours in inaccessible sites such as the back of the eye and pituitary. Their limitation is the technology required to produce a beam for routine medical use.

Biological actions of ionizing radiation

Ionizing radiation causes damage to cellular DNA both directly and indirectly through toxic-free radicals produced from the interaction of radiation with water within the cell. This results in single and double strand breaks in the DNA and unless repair occurs these will accumulate resulting in reproductive death of the cell.

Other factors which are important in the response to radiation include:

Oxygenation

Hypoxic tissues are considered relatively radioresistant. Fractionation of treatment allows reoxygenation to occur between each treatment as the tumour shrinks and blood flow improves.

Repopulation

Both tumour tissue and normal tissues continue to divide during a course of radiotherapy and there is even some evidence to suggest that repopulation may increase during this time as cells are lost. Gaps of days between radiotherapy treatment should therefore be avoided wherever possible to prevent significant repopulation undoing any effects from irradiation in the previous days.

Repair

Much of the damage produced by X-rays and gamma rays is not sufficient to kill the cell immediately and if repaired the cell can retain its viability. This capacity in normal tissues is relied on to establish differential cell kill between tumour and normal cells.

Redistribution

With redistribution within the cell cycle, radiosensitivity varies as cells progress through the cell cycle being maximum during the periods of active DNA synthesis in late G1 and S phases and least during G2 and early G1.

There is a spectrum of radiosensitivity for both tumour and normal cell types. Few if any tumours are truly radioresistant although some may require a larger dose of radiation to achieve the same effect as others. There is also a wide spectrum of sensitivity in normal tissues.

Particular care is required with certain normal tissues when delivering irradiation:

- CNS tissue has a relatively low threshold for damage and has little or no capacity for repair. Radiation damage to the CNS is therefore often irreversible and can result in catastrophic morbidity if, for example, necrosis of the spinal cord or brain stem results.
- The small bowel is also relatively sensitive and doses well below those required to sterilize an epithelial tumour will cause serious damage.
- The lens of the eye will develop cataract after exposure to only small doses and must therefore be carefully shielded whenever possible.
- Bladder and rectum are often dose-limiting tissues when treating pelvic tumours.
- Lung damage can result which if involving a large volume of lung can cause considerable respiratory distress and even death.

The balance between causing serious normal tissue damage and curing a malignant tumour is termed the 'therapeutic ratio' and is the major limitation to the success of radiotherapy in achieving local cure of malignant tumours.

Clinical use of radiotherapy

The patient attending for radiotherapy treatment will pass through a series of steps to ensure that treatment is given as accurately and safely as possible. These include:

- Patient positioning and immobilization
- Tumour localization.
- Treatment planning.
- Verification.
- Treatment.

Positioning of a patient is very important in order to enable an X-ray beam to reach a certain site. This is particularly the case in the head and neck region where small changes in the position of the neck or chin can greatly affect the tissues included in an X-ray beam. In order to be able to reproduce a particular position accurately some form of immobilization may be designed such as a plastic head shell to hold the head in a fixed position.

Tumour localization may be achieved by simple clinical examination as in the case of a skin tumour, plain X-rays, e.g. a bone metastasis, or CT scan for tumours in the thorax, abdomen or pelvis. Alongside this it is important to identify vital structures to be avoided such as the spinal cord or kidney. Identification of the area to be treated and structures to be avoided has to be related to the direction of an X-ray beam on that site. This is achieved usually by indelible skin marks placed at the time of taking the localization X-ray or scan.

Treatment planning involves designing the optimal arrangement of X-ray beams in order to cover the treatment area as evenly as possible while avoiding structures around it. At its simplest level this may be a single direct X-ray beam on a skin tumour; for internal tumours a more complex arrangement of two, three or four X-ray beams approaching from different directions may be required. Treatment plans of multiple beams are drawn up using computerized data describing the characteristics of the beam and enabling rapid addition of their effects at a point.

Verification entails ensuring that the treatment plan can be translated back to the patient in the defined treatment position. This is usually done on a machine called a treatment simulator which reproduces precisely the movements of the treatment machine but produces only a diagnostic X-ray beam so that an X-ray picture of the proposed treatment beam can be taken.

Further verification may also be performed when the actual treatment is started, particularly if complex beam shapes or lead shielding are to be employed. Megavoltage images can be taken. Their disadvantage is that because they interact in a different manner to low energy X-rays there is no differential absorption between bone and soft tissue.

Treatment only proceeds once it is certain that the defined area to be treated can be encompassed using the planned X-ray beams. During treatment the patient will be continually monitored by the radiographers and seen regularly by the medical staff. Specific additional measurements of radiation exposure may be taken using dosemeters placed on vital areas such as the eye or testes and further verification X-rays may be taken during the course of treatment.

Treatment duration

There is considerable variation in the dose and duration of radiotherapy treatment given to patients which can create considerable confusion even among radiotherapists. Neither the total number of treatments nor the total dose given are necessarily a guide to the biological dose of radiation delivered. There are three components to biological radiation dose:

1. Total dose.
2. Number of treatments (fractions) that dose is given in.
3. Overall time of treatment.

   The following general principles can be applied:

1. The same total dose given in a short time or fewer fractions has greater effect than the same dose given over a longer time in many fractions.
2. Fraction size is an important determinant of normal tissue damage; small fractions minimize normal tissue effects – but it follows from (1) that, if used, they demand a longer course of treatment with a higher total dose to have the same effect.
3. Overall treatment time is important in achieving tumour control. Delays and interruptions in a course of treatment should be avoided as should overall treatment times of greater than 6 to 7 weeks.

   The unit of radiation dose used is the Gray which is a measure of absorbed energy (1 Gray = 1 Joule per kilogram). This has replaced the rad but the conversion is simple: 1 Gray = 100 rads. In some centres in order to keep the actual numbers the same, doses are described in centigray since 1 cGy = 1 rad.

   Precise radiation schedules vary from centre to centre and between individual clinicians, however some generalizations can be made. A fundamental difference lies between palliative and radical doses.

   Radical treatments require high doses of radiation to eliminate tumour but are divided into smaller fractions to minimize side effects and remain within the tolerance of normal tissues. Examples of radical schedules include:

*   60 to 65 Gy in 30 to 32 fractions in 6 to 6.5 weeks.
*   55 Gy in 20 fractions in 4 weeks.
*   50 Gy in 15 fractions in 3 weeks.

   Palliative treatments require short schedules with few acute side effects. The ideal palliative treatment is a single dose and many centres use this routinely, while others treat over 1 to 2 weeks. Examples include:

*   8 to 10 Gy in a single dose.
*   20 Gy in 5 daily fractions over 1 week.

- 30 Gy in 10 daily fractions over 2 weeks.

Side effects of radiotherapy

The toxicity of radiotherapy is divided into two distinct groups: the early effects which occur during treatment and the late effects which come on months or years following treatment.

Early effects

These develop during treatment usually in the second to third week of a course of radical irradiation. They may be divided as follows:

1. Non-specific effects – many patients feel tired and lack energy during treatment. There may be many factors in addition to radiation exposure to account for this, including depression, anxiety, travelling daily to treatment and concomitant medication.
2. Specific local effects related to the area being treated. It is important to note that areas outside the irradiation field do not exhibit acute toxicity. Examples are shown in Table 5.1 together with suggested treatment. As a general principle these are all self-limiting effects which resolve spontaneously after treatment, their pathogenesis being related to temporary loss of cell division in an epithelial surface.

Table 5.1

Site	Effect	Treatment
Skin	Erythema leading if severe to desquamation	Minimal; avoid irritants, trauma. Aqueous or weak hydrocortisone cream
Bowel	Diarrhoea/colic	Low residue diet Codeine or loperamide
Bladder	Frequency/dysuria	Exclude infection
Scalp	Hair loss	Order wig in advance. Will regrow after palliative but not radical doses
Mouth/pharynx	Mucositis	Avoid irritants. Treat candidiasis. Topical chlorhexidine or benzydamine

Late effects

These are potentially the most serious effects of treatment since unlike the acute effects they are not self-limiting and indeed tend to be progressive and irreversible. They arise due to loss of stem cell recovery potential and progressive damage to small blood vessels resulting in their occlusion (endarteritis obliterans).

Fortunately in practice they are rare but any radical treatment dose will carry a risk of late damage becoming manifest in the months and years ahead. They are not usually seen before 6 months after treatment but there is an ongoing risk which is never entirely lost.

Finally the risk of inducing second malignancy should be considered. In practice this is exceedingly rare and invariably outweighed by risk from the established malignancy for which radiation is given. A clear pattern is recognized with leukaemia or lymphoma seen in the first few years after exposure reaching a peak incidence around 3 years and not seen after 10 years. In contrast solid tumours have an increasing risk with time, are rarely seen before 10 years and may occur 30 years or more after exposure.

The greatest risk may be associated with low dose exposure and there are many examples after treatment of benign disease such as tinea capitis, goitre and ankylosing spondylitis. After therapeutic radiation the risk is small but there is some evidence that this may be increased in patients who receive combined modality treatment with the addition of chemotherapy. This has recently become apparent in long-term survivors of lymphoma treatments in whom the risk after 20 years of a second tumour is around 15 per cent.

Table 5.2

Site	Effect	Treatment
Skin	Fibrosis, telangiectasia. Rarely necrosis	Usually none
Bowel	Stricture, perforation. Bleeding, fistulae	If severe resection of affected segment
Bladder	Fibrosis causing frequency, haematuria. Fistulae	If severe surgical resection
CNS	Myelitis causing paraplegia. Cerebral necrosis	None
Lung	Fibrosis	None

Radiation protection

Indiscriminant use of radiation is dangerous. There are strict regulations surrounding its use for medical purposes to ensure that exposure to staff, visitors and patients is kept to an absolute minimum. This is achieved by physical separation and protection from the sources of radiation and subsequent monitoring of exposure in those at particular risk.

Separation and protection

Radiotherapy machines are localized in one area or even in a separate hospital. Their design incorporates shielding of scattered radiation to produce a defined beam, the penetration and qualities of which are carefully measured and maintained. They are housed within a room designed to contain the radiation, using lead barriers within the walls for low energy beams and thick high density concrete walls for high energy beams.

Similarly, radioisotopes are stored under carefully controlled conditions in a radiation safe and administered to the patient in a designated area again designed to contain any radiation exposure. Patients having implants or high levels of radioiodine will be isolated in single rooms which have additional shielding to prevent radiation reaching other areas of the ward, and staff are given strict time limits to be spent with the patient. Visitors are usually not permitted while there are high levels of radioactivity present.

Radiation monitoring

All staff involved in the direct care of patients receiving radiation treatment will be designated as workers who require regular monitoring for radiation exposure. The mainstay of monitoring is the film badge worn by these staff which when processed will detect those who may have been inadvertently exposed to radiation. There are clearly defined exposure limits for adults within which all personnel must remain. All departments must have local rules regarding the handling and use of radiation sources and staff must be fully acquainted with these.

It is important to keep the dangers of radiation as used under controlled medical conditions in context, while not relaxing the rules governing its use. There is no evidence that hospital workers are at greater risk than the general population from malignant disease. The entire population is exposed to levels of background radiation and many other common daily activities carry a greater risk than low level exposure, for example it has been estimated that all of the following carry a one in a million risk of death:

- Driving for 65 miles.
- Flying in civil aircraft for 400 miles.
- Smoking less than one cigarette.
- Drinking half a bottle of wine.

6

Principles of chemotherapy

Cancer chemotherapy is the treatment of malignant disease with drugs rather than radiation or surgical removal. The drugs used are often highly toxic since they are rarely, if ever, selective for cancer cells and are therefore best given within an oncology unit by those experienced in their use.

Chemotherapy agents

Cancer chemotherapy agents act upon cell division interfering with normal cell replication. They can be broadly classified into five main groups (Fig. 6.1):

Antimetabolites

These function at the level of DNA synthesis interfering with the incorporation of nucleic acid bases (cytosine, thymine, adenine and guanine). Two types of drug are currently available:

- Drugs based on chemical modification of a nucleic acid so that the

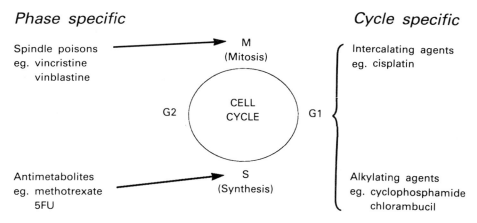

Fig. 6.1 Classification of cytotoxic drugs according to their action on the cell cycle.

drug rather than the true nucleic acid is incorporated into the DNA thereby preventing accurate replication of the complementary base sequence, e.g. 5-fluorouracil (5FU) or cytosine arabinoside
- Inhibition of the reduction of folic acid from its inactive dihydrofolate form to the active tetrahydrofolate. Folic acid is essential for the transfer of methyl groups in DNA synthesis. Methotrexate acts in this way.

Alkylating agents

These directly interfere with the DNA double strand of base pairs by chemically reacting with the structure forming methyl cross-bridges. These then prevent the two DNA strands coming apart in mitosis to form daughter DNA fragments and division therefore fails. Drugs in this group include cyclophosphamide, chlorambucil, melphelan and the nitrosoureas BCNU and CCNU.

Intercalating agents

These act in a similar way to the alkylating agents but rather than directly forming cross-strands in the DNA molecule they bind between the base pair molecules, i.e. binding adenine to thymidine and cytosine to guanine again preventing the DNA double strand from dividing in order to replicate and thereby stopping cell division.

Spindle poisons

These act by preventing spindle formation which is essential in the sorting and moving of chromosomes following replication at the end of mitosis. The drugs in this group are the vinca alkaloids; vincristine, vinblastine and vindesine.

Other agents

Other drugs which are active whose precise mode of action is unknown include mitomycin C and bleomycin.

Because of their mode of action certain drugs require cells to be in specific phases of the cell cycle to have any effect. For example, those acting on synthesis of DNA will only act on cells actively synthesizing at the time they are exposed to the drug. Cytotoxic drugs are therefore further classified into:

- Phase specific acting only in a specific phase of the cell cycle, e.g. antimetabolites during 'S' phase and vinca alkaloids in 'M' phase.
- Cycle specific which require that cells are only dividing and passing through the cell cycle rather than being in the resting Go phase. These include the alkylating agents.

Efficacy and toxicity of chemotherapy

Although in principle all cycling cells should be sensitive to drugs acting upon their replication, in practice chemotherapy for most cancers is only modestly effective. This is due to a variety of reasons related to drug delivery to the cell and activation or deactivation within the target cells. Precise indications for the use of chemotherapy are detailed in the following chapters but in general the common malignant diseases can be broadly classified into three groups: those extremely sensitive to chemotherapy where this is the treatment of choice; those with modest sensitivity where chemotherapy may play a part in their management but usually in combination with other treatment as an adjuvant or for recurrent disease; and finally those where chemotherapy is rarely of value. Examples of the classification are given in Table 6.1.

Table 6.1 Sensitivity to chemotherapy

Group 1 *Highly sensitive*	Group 2 *Modest sensitivity*	Group 3 *Low sensitivity*
Leukaemias	Breast	Prostate
Lymphomas	Colorectal	Kidney
Germ cell tumours	Bladder	Primary brain tumour
Small cell lung cancer	Ovary	Adult sarcomas
Myeloma		Cervix
Neuroblastoma		Endometrium
Wilm's tumour		
Embryonal rhabdomyosarcoma		

Response and survival

In describing the efficacy of chemotherapeutic agents there are clearly defined response criteria as follows:

Complete response (CR) – complete resolution of all clinically detectable disease for a period of at least 1 month.

Partial response (PR) – a reduction in tumour dimensions of at least 50 per cent maintained for at least 1 month. The dimension usually referred to is the maximum diameter of a tumour mass.

Stable disease (SD) – no change or a response which is less than a partial response or progression less than a 25 per cent increase in measurable disease during the period of observation.

Progressive disease (PD) – an increase in measurable disease of at least 25 per cent during the period of observation, or the development of any new lesions.

It is important to interpret with care response data derived from clinical trials. Unless an agent or drug combination achieves a complete response in a significant proportion of patients then it is unlikely to have any impact on overall survival when used to treat that disease in the general population. Partial responses may be of value in delaying progression of a disease but since they represent only a very small decrement in total cancer cell burden significant effects on overall survival are unlikely.

With this in mind performance status and quality of life measures are becoming an increasingly important measure of the efficacy of cancer treatment. Numerous scales of performance status have been devised, the most widespread of which is perhaps the Karnofsky scale shown in Table 6.2. Quality of life measures are more complex and usually involve some form of structured questionnaire into the patient's activities and interests.

Table 6.2 Karnofsky scale for performance status

100	Normal; no complaints; no evidence of disease
90	Able to carry on normal activities' minor signs or symptoms
80	Normal activity with effort; some signs or symptoms of disease
70	Cares for self; unable to carry on normal activity or do active work
60	Requires occasional assistance but able to care for most needs
50	Requires considerable assistance and frequent medical care
40	Disabled; requires special care and assistance
30	Severely disabled; hospitalization indicated although death not imminent
20	Very sick; hospitalization necessary; active supportive treatment necessary
10	Moribund; fatal processes progressing rapidly
0	Dead

Clinical use of chemotherapy

Cytotoxic drugs may be given as single agents or more usually in combination with other cytotoxic drugs. The major limitation in using these agents, lies in their toxicity to normal tissues. Because they are all non-specific in their action both malignant and normal cells are damaged when exposed to a cytotoxic drug. When used within their defined dose limits the normal cells will recover and it is the need for this window of normal cell recovery that results in the typical intermittent scheduling of these agents most being given at 3 to 4 weekly intervals.

Common limiting toxicities are bone marrow suppression, bowel toxicity, and renal and neurological damage. Agents for which these are major limiting factors are shown in Table 6.3.

Combination chemotherapy

For many conditions combinations of drugs are used. This results from a balance of adding together modestly active agents to give greater overall activity and spreading different toxicities. Combinations are also designed to incorporate drugs from different classes thereby attacking cells with

Table 6.3   Major toxicities for chemotherapeutic agents

Bone marrow – all drugs in particular

Vinblastine	Cyclophosphamide
Etoposide	Melphelan
Carboplatin	Ifosphamide

Bowel	*Renal*	*Neurological*
Melphelan	Methotrexate	Cisplatin
Cisplatin	Cisplatin	Vincristine
5FU	Ifosphamide	Ifosphamide
Methotrexate		

Others
Adriamycin – cardiac
Cyclophosphamide – bladder

*In practice bone marrow toxicity is becoming less important as a limiting toxicity as techniques for bone marrow support such as autologous marrow or peripheral stem cell transplantation become available.

both phase and cycle specific agents with the intent of targeting as many cells in the population as possible. An example of spreading limiting toxicities is shown in Table 6.4 with CHOP used for non-Hodgkin's lymphoma.

Table 6.4   Drugs in CHOP

Drug	Action	Main toxicity
Cyclophosphamide	Alkylating agent	Bone marrow
		Bladder
Adriamycin	Intercalating	Bone marrow
		Cardiac
Vincristine	Spindle poison	Neurological
		(peripheral neuropathy)
Prednisolone	Unknown	Fluid retention
		Gastric irritation

Administration

Chemotherapy should only be administered in specialized units with the experience and support to do so safely. Most of the agents used can be harmful if there is continuous contact with the skin and even more so if accidentally ingested through contamination of hands and work surfaces. Agents should therefore be prepared by a specialized chemotherapy pharmacist under strictly controlled conditions and gloves should be worn by the clinical staff when administering the drugs.

Prior to administration all patients should have a full blood count measured. As a general rule chemotherapy should only be given if the following parameters are met:

- Haemoglobin > 10 g/dl – although this is rarely a limiting factor and it is acceptable to proceed at lower levels and transfuse if necessary.
- Total white count > $3.0 \times 10^9/l$ – or total neutrophil count > 1.5.
- Platelets > $80 \times 10^9/l$.

For certain drugs renal function must also be carefully checked prior to administration. It is not usually sufficient to rely on serum urea or creatinine and a creatinine clearance or EDTA clearance should be performed. This applies in particular to the following:

- Cisplatin.
- Methotrexate (particularly at high doses).
- Ifosfamide.
- Carboplatin.

Chemotherapy drugs may be given orally, by intravenous or intramuscular bolus injection or by intravenous infusion. Examples of these are shown in Table 6.5.

Table 6.5 Routes of administration

Oral	IV injection	Infusion
Chlorambucil	Cyclophosphamide	Cisplatin
Busulphan	Methotrexate	Carboplatin
Melphelan (ld)	5FU	Mitozantrone
Procarbazine	Adriamycin	Ifosfamide
Etoposide	Vincristine	Methotrexate (hd)
	Vinblastine	Melphelan (hd)

ld = low dose. hd = high dose.

Many chemotherapy drugs are extremely irritant when injected outside a vein and extreme care must be taken during intravenous injections. These should be performed ideally by experienced staff working in a dedicated chemotherapy administration unit. Large visible veins should be chosen as far as possible and it is safest to administer the drugs into a running intravenous drip.

If extravasation does occur then there should be clear guidelines for its management. The following principles apply:

- The chemotherapy injection or infusion must be stopped immediately.
- The cannula is left *in situ* and the area flushed with saline.
- Ice packs may be applied and some recommend local steroids or hyaluronidase.

In severe cases with irritant drugs such as adriamycin or epirubicin there may be extensive soft tissue damage as shown in Figure 6.2, particularly if the problem is not identified immediately and action taken.

Fig. 6.2   Severe soft tissue damage following extravasation of chemotherapy given intravenously into the back of the hand.

Liaison with a plastic surgery unit for such eventualities is of great value. Occasionally damage may be such as to require surgical repair.

Avoiding side effects

As a general rule side effects are best anticipated and prevented. Chemo-therapy agents vary in their emetic potential but all may cause nausea and some severe vomiting. Anti-emetics should therefore be considered for all but the most gentle of agents. A three-stage anti-emetic policy will work for most patients.

Emetic potential of common chemotherapy agents

The following, used as single agents, rarely cause significant nausea and either anti-emetics are not required or simple oral agents are sufficient:

- Chlorambucil.
- Vincristine/vinblastine.

Other drugs or combinations fall into the groups shown in Table 6.6.

Table 6.6

Low	Moderate	High
5FU	Cyclophosphamide	Cisplatin
Bleomycin	Methotrexate	Carboplatin
	Adriamycin	Ifosphamide
Etoposide	Mitozantrone	Mustine

Table 6.7   Antiemetic policy for cytotoxic drugs

Low potential schedules:
   Metoclopramide 10 mg or prochlorperazine 12.5 mg intravenously with
   chemotherapy

Moderately emetogenic schedules:
   Dexamethasone 8 mg
   Metoclopramide 10 mg } intravenously with chemotherapy
followed by dexamethasone 2 mg tds
             metoclopramide 10 mg tds } orally for 2 to 3 days

Highly emetogenic schedules:
   Dexamethasone 8 mg
   High dose metoclopramide
   (2 to 3 mg/kg by infusion) } with chemotherapy
followed by dexamethasone 2 mg tds
             metoclopramide 10 mg tds } orally for 2 to 3 days
or
   Dexamethasone 8 mg
   Ondansetron 8 mg } intravenously with chemotherapy
followed by, if necessary, ondansetron 4 mg daily for 2 days

The use of anti-emetic drugs varies considerably among different units. A simple anti-emetic protocol is shown in Table 6.7.

Anticipatory nausea and vomiting may be a particular problem for some patients when they experience symptoms with any visit to the hospital without exposure to the drugs. Lorazepam may be helpful in these instances. It is also often easier for inpatients to receive chemotherapy in the evening when they may have added sedation and sleep through the administration.

Other side effects must also be anticipated and steps taken to prevent them. For example:

- Diarrhoea (e.g. cisplatin) – prescribe codeine phosphate.
- Mucositis (e.g. 5FU, methotrexate) – use regular chlorhexadine and benzydamine mouthwashes.

Scheduling

Chemotherapy schedules vary from simple single oral drugs to complex multiple drug regimes. The design of drug schedules is based on a consideration of the effects on both normal tissues and the tumour cells.

Normal tissues are inevitably damaged by chemotherapy agents. Particularly sensitive are the dividing cells of the bone marrow and mucosal epithelial cells lining the oropharynx, gut and bladder. The general principle of scheduling chemotherapy is that each successive course should only be given when repairable damage from the previous drug exposure has been repaired. Fortunately both bone marrow and epithelial lining cells have a large capacity for absorbing and recovering from damage to them and usually do so within 2 to 3 weeks. On this basis most chemotherapy is given at 3 to 4 weekly intervals.

Damage to tumour cells may depend on both the absolute levels of drug which can be achieved within them and the duration of exposure. In order to achieve the maximum levels possible a fine line may be drawn between serious side effects and maximizing tumour cell kill. In some circumstances where there is evidence that very high doses of drugs not normally tolerated will achieve more, e.g. acute leukaemia, then bone marrow may be removed prior to chemotherapy and stored to be used as an autograft once high dose therapy has been given. These are at present, however, exceptional procedures.

In order to achieve maximum levels for a suitable duration a knowledge of the pharmacokinetics of the drug is important. Drugs with short half-lives may have a greater effect when given by infusion or in divided doses, e.g. 5FU.

The design of chemotherapy drug schedules is often a combination of elegant hypothesis, serendipity and pragmatism. However, when assessing the results of chemotherapy trials and translating them into general oncological practice careful attention to the drug dosing and scheduling is important. There is some evidence that patients who fail to receive full doses of drugs at the designated minimum intervals have a reduced benefit from the treatment and this is a strong argument for chemotherapy being managed only in experienced units familiar with the complications and tolerance for each schedule.

Experimental chemotherapy

The chemotherapy drugs and combination regimes which are widely used in routine oncological practice today have arisen out of carefully designed and regulated drug development programmes. From discovery of a promising new drug in the laboratory a lengthy and expensive period of evaluation starting with animal pharmacology and toxicology studies and ending in successful drug marketing has to be embarked on. The clinical studies within which new drugs may be given are outlined below.

1. Phase 1 studies in which the new agent is first tried in patients. Such agents are offered only to patients for whom there is no other recognized effective treatment and who may wish to try other drugs in the slim hope of benefit. In phase 1 studies activity against the tumour is not an end-point but these studies are designed to assess the maximum tolerated doses and define the toxicity profile in humans.
2. Phase 2 studies are the earliest studies in which anti-tumour activity is sought, giving the drug in doses and schedules defined from the phase 1 studies to patients who have failed previous conventional therapy or for whom there may be no effective recognized treatment.
3. Phase 3 studies in which, having established activity in phase 2, the new agent is compared with the standard best treatment (or, if there

is none, with placebo) in a large prospective randomized trial. Large numbers of patients are entered into such trials in order to achieve statistically robust results and most of these studies are therefore multicentre studies.

Only following satisfactory passage through the above steps is a drug incorporated in the routine treatment of cancer; this may be many years after the first identification of the compound and will be followed by further evaluation of the drug to establish its full potential and application in adjuvant and primary treatment and its role in palliation both alone and in combination. Its toxicity in wider use must also be continuously monitored and notified (post-marketing surveillance).

7

Lung cancer

Epidemiology

There are 41 000 new cases of lung cancer and 40 000 deaths are registered in the UK per annum. It is the major cause of cancer mortality in this country with a peak incidence of 60–70 years. It is three times more common in men in whom it is most common cancer. The mortality in men is declining, but increasing in women due to changes in smoking habits in recent decades.

Aetiology

The majority of cases can be attributed to exposure of the bronchial epithelium to inhaled carcinogens. Cytogenetic studies have shown loss of a tumour suppressor gene on part of the short arm of chromosome 3 in some cases of small cell lung cancer (SCLC), although the disease does not have a hereditary component.

There is a strong causal relationship between smoking and lung cancer with 90 per cent of cases attributable to the use of tobacco. The bronchial tree and alveoli are directly exposed to the inhaled smoke and it is the hydrocarbon carcinogens such as benzpyrene liberated by the combustion of tar that are responsible rather than nicotine. These lead to metaplasia of the bronchial epithelium from a columnar pattern to a squamous one, eventually leading to dysplasia and carcinoma *in situ*. The risk of developing lung cancer is related to the duration and intensity of smoking, increasing with the rise in number of cigarettes or weight of tobacco smoked per day, increasing tar content, shorter cigarette stubs and use of non-filter brands. The tumours tend to be found adjacent to the larger airways of the lung comprising mainly squamous cell carcinoma (SCC) and SCLC. Recent evidence suggests that passive smoking leads to an increased risk if the spouse smokes 20 cigarettes per day or more. The lung cancer risk declines towards that of non-smokers after 10–20 years of abstinence although there is a persistent risk in those who have smoked more than 20 per day.

It is important to elicit a history of occupational asbestos exposure in patients with lung cancer as they may be eligible for industrial injuries compensation. The carcinogenic potential of asbestos is synergistic with that of tobacco smoking and of the many types of asbestos the blue variant is the most powerful carcinogen. Asbestos-induced cancers are more common in the lower lobes, usually SCC, and may be multicentric.

During the 19th century, cobalt miners in Eastern Europe were noted to have a very high mortality from lung cancer due to high levels of radon gas released from the granite-bearing rocks by the radioactive decay of naturally occurring uranium, which in turn led to high doses of radiation to the bronchial tree and eventual malignant transformation. There is evidence that the level of radon in dwellings may account for a small proportion of deaths from lung cancer in the UK each year, and an increased incidence of lung cancer has also been noted in patients who have had previous spinal irradiation for ankylosing spondylitis.

Nickel, arsenic and chromates have all been implicated as causes of lung cancer.

Tuberculous scars, subpleural blebs/bullae or the site of a previous pulmonary embolus may occasionally account for peripheral carcinomas, particularly adenocarcinoma.

Pathology

Macroscopically, lung cancers arise within the bronchial epithelium and therefore usually have an endobronchial component. They may be multifocal and may arise anywhere in the bronchial tree, although SCC and SCLC often arise centrally in the larger airways while adenocarcinomas usually arise peripherally, particularly at the apices. Central necrosis leads to cavitation in the larger tumours.

Microscopically, lung cancers may be divided into:

1. Squamous cell carcinoma (50 per cent) – this may be preceded by the stepwise progression from squamous metaplasia to dysplasia followed by carcinoma *in situ* and frankly invasive cancer. The tumour cells have the morphology of squamous epithelial cells, stain for keratin and intercellular bridges are visible under the electron microscope, these features being more evident in well-differentiated tumours.
2. Small cell carcinoma (25 per cent) – these arise from the Kulchitsky cells of the basal layer of the bronchial epithelium and are characterized histologically by small, uniform cells containing neurosecretory granules and staining for neurone specific enolase (NSE) reflecting their origin from cells derived from the neural crest of the foetus. The ectopic production of peptides and hormones will be reflected in their immunocytochemical staining. There are several subtypes, the best known of which is the oat cell carcinoma which is composed of sheets of fusiform cells.
3. Adenocarcinoma (15 per cent) – the tumour cells stain for mucin reflecting their glandular origin and may be arranged in an acinar pattern.
4. Large cell anaplastic (10 per cent) – these are poorly differentiated

and cannot be recognized under the light microscope as belonging to any of the other subgroups. Clear cell and giant cell tumours are included in this group (see Rare tumours).

Natural history

The pattern of growth of a lung cancer is related to the histological subtype. The anaplastic carcinomas are the most rapid growing, while adenocarcinomas grow slowly and may be seen to have been present over several years prior to diagnosis. SCLC has a propensity to early and widespread metastatic dissemination with 80–90 per cent having spread beyond the thorax by the time of diagnosis.

Lung cancer spreads circumferentially and longitudinally along the bronchus of origin eventually leading to bronchial occlusion which causes lobar or segmental pulmonary collapse due to resorption of air distal to the tumour. Stasis of pulmonary secretions in turn leads to secondary infection manifesting as pneumonia and occasionally lung abscess and empyema. Proximally the tumour may extend to the carina and trachea while distally it may reach the visceral pleura from where it may invade the chest wall, interlobar fissures or pleural space resulting in a blood-stained exudative pleural effusion. A pneumothorax may result from a tumour which breaches the visceral pleura and allows a direct connection between the pleural space and the bronchial tree. Mediastinal structures such as the oesophagus, pericardium, heart and great vessels and occasionally the vertebral bodies and diaphragm may be invaded.

The tumour frequently involves the regional lymphatics spreading to ipsilateral peribronchial and hilar nodes, followed by subcarinal, contralateral hilar, paratracheal and supraclavicular nodes.

Lung cancer has a propensity to disseminate widely via the bloodstream and virtually any site may be involved. There is an unusual and unexplained involvement of the adrenal glands in a high proportion of cases. Other common sites include the liver, skeleton, brain (especially SCLC), skin and contralateral lung.

Symptoms

A small proportion of patients will present with no symptoms, having been diagnosed on a chest X-ray either as part of a routine screen or as part of the investigation of another disease. Most, however, present due to intrathoracic symptoms.

Cough is due to bronchial irritation by the tumour and is often unproductive unless associated with secondary infection. Bronchoalveolar tumours (see Rare tumours, p. 60) characteristically result in the expectoration of large quantities of mucoid sputum. The cough will have a 'bovine' character if there is also a vocal cord palsy.

Haemoptysis varying in severity from slight streaking of the sputum with blood to frank haemorrhage is common where there is a large intrabronchial component to the tumour with mucosal ulceration.

Dyspnoea reflects a deficiency in pulmonary ventilation due to a restrictive defect (e.g. pleural effusion, diffuse parenchymal infiltration), obstructive defect (e.g. bronchial obstruction by tumour or secondary infection) or a combination of the two. It will first be noticed on mild exertion, progressing to dyspnoea at rest.

Chest pain may be pleuritic or aching in nature and localized to the involved hemithorax, reflecting pleural involvement by tumour, secondary infection of the pleura or direct invasion of the chest wall.

Recurrent chest infections are a common presenting feature and carcinoma of the lung should be considered in anyone of the appropriate age who has had recurrent chest infections for no apparent cause or an infection which has failed to resolve following one or more courses of the appropriate antibiotic.

Dysphagia may result from extrinsic compression from the primary tumour, particularly if the tumour is arising from the left main bronchus as the oesophagus is a close anatomical relation posteriorly. A large mass of involved lymph nodes (usually subcarinal) should also be considered as a cause.

A hoarse voice suggests invasion of the recurrent laryngeal nerve, giving rise to a vocal cord paralysis which in turn results in a hoarse voice and 'bovine' cough due to failure to adduct the vocal cords. Indirect laryngoscopy in the clinic or visualization of the cords at bronchoscopy will be diagnostic.

Tumours arising at the lung apex may cause nerve root pain as they lead to direct invasion of the T1 nerve root leading to pain radiating down the ipsilateral arm to the medial aspect of the forearm, and may lead to infiltration of the spinal cord itself.

Non-specific extrathoracic symptoms include anorexia, weight loss, malaise and lethargy.

Signs

No physical signs at all may be elicited, particularly in those presenting without symptoms after a routine chest X-ray. Pulmonary collapse and/or consolidation is the most frequent finding. Examination of the hands frequently reveals clubbing, characterized by an increase in nail convexity in the transverse and longitudinal planes, loss of the nail fold angle and sponginess of the nail bed on compression of the nail. There may be nicotine staining of the fingers.

The supraclavicular lymph nodes should be checked as these are the only palpable nodes that are in continuity with the regional lymphatics.

The syndrome of superior vena caval obstruction deserves special mention (see Chapter 22).

Involvement of the cervical sympathetic nerves leads to Horner's syndrome characterized by partial ptosis, miosis (pupillary constriction), enophthalmos (indrawing of the globe of the eye relative to the orbit) and anhydrosis (loss of sweating on the ipsilateral side of the face). The ipsilateral hand may be warmer due to vasodilation, and there will be wasting of the small muscles of the hand as these are partly innervated by the T1 nerve root.

A small proportion will present with one or more of a variety of clinical syndromes which are unassociated with metastases. These are the so-called non-metastatic manifestations of malignancy (Table 7.1).

Other signs will depend on the tumour burden and sites of spread.

Table 7.1 Non-metastatic manifestations of lung cancer

Cutaneous	Dermatomyositis
	Acanthosis nigricans
	Erythema gyratum ripens
	Hypertrichosis languinosa
	Clubbing
	Hypertrophic pulmonary osteoarthropathy (HPOA)
	Scleroderma
	Herpes zoster
	Urticaria
Neuromuscular	Myositis
	Proximal myopathy
	Peripheral neuropathy
	Mononeuritis multiplex
	Cortical degeneration
	Progressive multifocal leucoencephalopathy
	Transverse myelitis
	Cerebellar degeneration
	Eaton–Lambert myasthenic syndrome
Ectopic hormone production	Hypokalaemia and water retention (ADH)
	Hyperpigmentation and hypokalaemic alkalosis (ACTH)
	Hypercalcaemia (PTH)
	Carcinoid (5HT)
	Hypoglycaemia (insulin-like peptides)
	Hyperglycaemia (glucagon, growth hormone)
	Gynaecomastia and testicular atrophy (gonadotrophins, HCG)
	Hypertension (renin)
Haematological	Anaemia (may be sideroblastic)
	Disseminated intravascular coagulation
	Eosinophilia
	Thrombocytosis
	Thrombocytopaenia
	Leucocytosis/leukaemoid picture
	Red cell aplasia
	Bone marrow plasmacytosis
Miscellaneous	Murantic endocarditis (may lead to systemic emboli)
	Membranous glomerulonephritis
	Hypouricaemia
	Hyperamylasaemia
	Migratory thrombophlebitis (Trousseau's syndrome)

Differential diagnosis

This includes:

1. Benign tumours – papilloma, hamartoma, carcinoid, fibroma, leio-myoma.
2. Other malignant primary tumours – mesothelioma, bronchial gland carcinomas, soft tissue sarcomas.
3. Metastases.
4. Non-neoplastic diseases, e.g. aspergilloma, chronic lung abscess, Wegener's granulomatosis, radiographic artefact, e.g. nipple shadow.

Investigations

A full blood count, liver function tests and serum calcium should be checked in all new patients. Additional investigations include the following.

Chest X-ray

This has the advantage of providing a relatively rapid, non-invasive, widely available means of ascertaining the position, size and number of tumours. For optimal assessment, a PA and lateral view should always be requested. Common features of lung cancer include a discrete opacity (Fig. 7.1a) which may be cavitating, hilar lymphadenopathy, pulmonary collapse, consolidation, and pleural effusion. Associated intrathoracic complications due to local invasion may be assessed, special care being taken to look for rib erosion in peripherally placed tumours (Fig. 7.1b). The hemidiaphragms should be inspected looking for excessive elevation – the right is usually slightly higher than the left due to the underlying liver. An elevated hemidiaphragm suggests palsy of the ipsilateral phrenic nerve, which in turn suggests mediastinal infiltration and therefore an inoperable tumour.

Sputum cytology

This is a rapid means of obtaining a tissue diagnosis with minimal patient inconvenience and distress, having the advantage of being suitable for outpatients while awaiting a definitive investigation such as a bronchoscopy. The sensitivity of the test increases with the number of sputum specimens collected and so at least three specimens are desirable. Samples should represent bronchial secretions rather than saliva and the best time for collection is early in the morning. Prior to collection, 5 ml of nebulized saline and physiotherapy may help a patient who has a non-productive cough. Central tumours are most likely to be detected in this way, particularly those associated with a large endobronchial component i.e. squamous carcinoma.

Bronchoscopy

This should be performed whenever active treatment is indicated. A fibre-optic bronchoscope is passed down the respiratory tract via the nose using topical anaesthesia, although rigid bronchoscopy under general anaesthesia is sometimes performed by the thoracic surgeon. Detailed anatomical information is gained regarding the precise location of the tumour within the bronchial tree which is of value when surgery or radiotherapy is contemplated; vocal cord palsy also may be confirmed on entry into the lower respiratory tract with the scope. Once visualized, the tumour can be biopsied or if the tumour is located too peripherally for the bronchoscope to reach it, saline can be injected and aspirated and the 'washings' sent for cytology; a small brush can be used to obtain 'brushings' from the epithelial lining of the bronchi. Bronchoscopy may also allow emergency procedures to be performed such as diathermy or laser of a bleeding tumour.

(a)

(b)

Fig. 7.1   (a) Early cancer appearing as a small opacity in the right lower zone. (b) Collapse and consolidation at the site of an apical cancer. Note deviation of the trachea to the side of the collapse, the narrowed intercostal spaces and erosion of the overlying ribs laterally.

CT scan

This is indicated whenever curative treatment is contemplated. It is the investigation of choice for detecting chest wall invasion, particularly in the case of apical tumours, and for detecting mediastinal lymphadenopathy, both of which individually are contraindications to surgical resection. The thorax is scanned to supplement the findings on plain X-rays and bronchoscopy, and the liver and adrenals are included for further staging information. A limited CT scan can also be used to assist percutaneous needle biopsy in those patients in whom a tissue diagnosis cannot be obtained by less invasive investigations.

Isotope bone scan

This is performed to exclude bone metastases.

Biopsy of palpable metastases

Biopsy or fine needle aspiration of palpable metastatic deposits such as a supraclavicular lymph node or a cutaneous nodule is a relatively atraumatic means of obtaining a tissue diagnosis.

Mediastinotomy/mediastinoscopy

These are invasive surgical investigations to determine whether the tumour is operable by allowing the surgeon to visualize and sample the mediastinal lymph nodes. Such procedures have been superseded by the CT scan.

Thoracotomy

This is the most invasive means of obtaining tumour tissue for histopathology, and is reserved for the very small proportion of patients who are not diagnosed after routine investigations. Unless the tumour has been shown to be inoperable during pre-operative assessment, the surgeon will aim to proceed to radical resection after frozen section has been performed, particularly for non-small cell cancer.

Lung function tests

These are performed to assess the patient's ventilatory capacity with regard to the compliance of the lungs and degree of airways obstruction and are only required prior to definitive lung resection as a guide to how disabled the patient would be post-operatively. A simpler guide is the patient's exercise tolerance – inability to climb a flight of stairs without stopping would be considered a contraindication to surgery.

Indirect laryngoscopy

This is indicated if the patient has an unexplained vocal abnormality and entails visualization of the position and mobility of the two vocal cords using a laryngeal mirror in the ENT clinic. Partial or complete palsy suggests pressure on the recurrent laryngeal nerve.

Staging

There is no formal staging system in routine clinical use. The TNM staging is complex and the reader is referred to a more specialized text. With SCLC, a two category staging system is used which correlates well with prognosis and serves as a guide to determining the most appropriate therapy in clinical trials:

1. Limited – extent of tumour as defined by physical examination and radiological investigations is confined to the ipsilateral hemithorax and ipsilateral supraclavicular nodes.
2. Extensive – defined as disease other than limited stage.

Management

Radical treatment of non-small cell lung cancer (NSCLC)
Surgery

Complete surgical excision is desirable and offers the best chance of cure although only about 25 per cent of patients will be suitable candidates. Surgery will involve either lobectomy or pneumonectomy depending on the site of the tumour, its size and the patient's respiratory reserve. Both procedures have a significant mortality of approximately 5 per cent and 10 per cent respectively. Only 25 per cent of those selected for radical resection will be cured due to either occult persistence of local disease or distant metastases at the time of surgery. The survival rate following surgery varies greatly from series to series but is in the region of 20–30 per cent at 5 years and reflects the selection criteria used by the surgeon to determine which patients undergo surgery and the skill of the surgeon concerned. Table 7.2 outlines the contraindications to surgery.

Radiotherapy

Comparisons of radiotherapy versus surgery have often been confounded by the majority of poor performance status patients being treated with radiotherapy. This is partly because radiotherapy has the advantage of treating tumours adjacent to or directly involving vital thoracic structures which cannot be sacrificed at operation. Five year survivals of 10–20 per cent are achieved. Pre-operative and post-operative radiotherapy has not produced any significant prolongation of survival and is not routinely practised.

Radical treatment of small cell lung cancer
Surgery

There is no place for radical surgery in the treatment of SCLC.

Table 7.2 Contraindications to radical surgery for lung cancer

Patient parameter	Pre-operative investigation
Poor lung function	Routine lung function testing
Phrenic nerve palsy	Diaphragmatic screening only if suspected
Recurrent laryngeal nerve palsy	Indirect laryngoscopy if any voice abnormality elicited
Invasion of trachea or other major thoracic structures which cannot be sacrificed, e.g. aorta heart, superior vena cava, oesophagus, vertebral bodies	Routine bronchoscopy and CT scan
Distant metastases	Routine liver function tests, alkaline phosphatase isotope bone scan and CT scan to include liver and adrenals. Perform other staging investigations if clinically indicated

Radiotherapy

As with surgery, radiotherapy has no role in the initial management of SCLC. It is, however, of value in decreasing the risk of intrathoracic recurrence in those with limited disease who have had a complete response to initial chemotherapy. Prophylactic cranial irradiation decreases the incidence of cerebral metastases but does not increase survival as many will relapse elsewhere and therefore its role is controversial.

Chemotherapy

The propensity for SCLC to disseminate early and its inherent chemosensitivity means that systemic treatment with chemotherapy is the most appropriate initial management. Objective responses in the order of 70–90 per cent have been reported for a variety of schedules, the active drugs being cisplatin, carboplatin, cyclophosphamide, ifosfamide, etoposide, vincristine, adriamycin and methotrexate. Complete responses of 30–40 per cent can be expected in limited disease, and 20–30 per cent in those with extensive disease. Median survival for untreated limited SCLC is only 14 weeks, falling to 7 weeks for extensive disease. Chemotherapy improves the median survival significantly to 12–18 months for limited disease and 9 months for extensive. There is no benefit in prolonging chemotherapy beyond 6 months in duration. Many of the long-term survivors develop cerebral metastases which may be due to chemotherapy drugs not crossing the blood-brain barrier in sufficient amounts to eradicate the tumour cells or due to seeding from sites of active disease elsewhere.

Palliative treatment of lung cancer

The priority of treatment is to relieve symptoms for the patient's remaining life-span with as little inconvenience and discomfort as possible.

Radiotherapy

Radiotherapy is very effective at relieving cough, chest pain and haemoptysis with palliation lasting for much of the patient's remaining life-span. Dyspnoea may be helped if it is due to bronchial obstruction. Large single doses of thoracic radiation are as effective as a more prolonged course (e.g. 10 fractions in 2 weeks) in terms of onset, quality and duration of response. Median survival of such patients is only 6 months, with a 1 year survival of 20 per cent falling to 5 per cent at 2 years. Palliative thoracic irradiation can be repeated if symptoms recur.

Chemotherapy

Low dose oral etoposide is useful in symptomatic SCLC patients with a low performance status and is given as an outpatient.

Other treatment modalities

Endobronchial laser therapy This is particularly useful for endobronchial tumours in relieving haemoptysis by permitting direct coagulation of the bleeding tumour and in relieving bronchial obstruction by acting as a cutting diathermy. It is frequently used in patients who have already received a maximal dose of radiation to the thorax.

Vocal cord apposition Teflon injection into the posterior two-thirds of the vocal cord leads to approximation of the vocal cords and is indicated for recurrent laryngeal nerve palsy when there is persistent aspiration of food and pharyngeal secretions into the bronchial tree leading to recurrent chest infections or respiratory distress.

Pleural/pericardial aspiration Drainage of pleural and pericardial effusions will rapidly relieve dyspnoea and sometimes any associated chest pain or dry cough.

Other medical measures include:

1. Antibiotics for chest infections.
2. Codeine linctus or methadone linctus as a cough suppressant.
3. Analgesics for chest pain.
4. Treatment of biochemical abnormalities resulting from non-metastatic manifestations.

Tumour-related complications

Complications can be divided into thoracic and extrathoracic. Thoracic complications include:

1. Pneumonia, pleural effusion, lung abscess, empyema, pneumothorax, massive pulmonary or pleural haemorrhage.
2. Atrial fibrillation, pericardial effusion.
3. Dysphagia, broncho-oesophageal fistula.
4. Sudden death from rupture of one of the great vessels.
5. Horner's syndrome, spinal cord compression.

Extrathoracic complications can be inferred from Table 7.1. Ectopic hormone production is most common with small cell carcinoma although SCC may produce a parathyroid hormone-like peptide leading to hypercalcaemia.

Treatment-related complications

Radiotherapy

Radiation oesophagitis is characterized by a feeling of retrosternal discomfort on swallowing food or fluids, particularly if hot or spicy, and beginning 2 weeks after commencing radiotherapy. Mucaine 10 ml tds before meals is of symptomatic benefit. Symptoms are rarely severe enough to interfere significantly with the patient's nutrition and usually subside within 2 weeks of finishing radiotherapy. Radiation pneumonitis has an acute phase beginning 6 weeks to 3 months after radiotherapy and is characterized by dry cough, fever, dyspnoea and chest pain. Radiologically there is a diffuse opacification of the lung corresponding to the applied radiation fields, which is often more severe than the symptoms would suggest. Mild cases resolve spontaneously but more severe cases will require treatment with a broad spectrum antibiotic together with prednisolone 20–40 mg daily. Some will progress to a chronic phase characterized by increasing pulmonary fibrosis leading to a restrictive defect and some degree of permanent respiratory compromise. The probability of pneumonitis can be minimized by using a small radiation dose per fraction and treating as small a lung volume as possible.

Surgery

Potential complications include:

1. Empyema due to infection within the pleural space.
2. Persistent bronchopleural fistula.
3. A decrease in respiratory reserve due to removal of lung tissue.
4. Discomfort related to the scar which may lead to an unremitting neuralgia.
5. Seeding of the tumour into the thoracotomy scar and subcutaneous tissues.

Chemotherapy

Most patients will experience alopecia as many of the drugs used for SCLC cause hair loss. Radiotherapy may increase the toxicity of drugs such as cyclophosphamide leading to pulmonary fibrosis and adriamycin leading to heart failure.

Prognosis

The prognosis from lung cancer remains poor and despite advances in surgery, radiotherapy and chemotherapy it has not changed for several decades. The three main poor prognostic factors include:

1. Advanced stage.
2. SCLC histology.
3. Poor performance status.

Patients with disease not amenable to radical therapy have a median survival of 6 months or less. Only about 5 per cent of SCLC patients survive 5 years compared with 10–20 per cent of those with NSCLC.

Screening

Several large prospective screening projects have been completed which have entailed regular chest X-rays or sputum cytology. These have not shown early detection by screening to improve survival in the screened population.

Prevention

Lung cancer is predominantly caused by smoking tobacco. Better health education, legislation to reduce cigarette advertising and punitive taxes on tobacco will decrease consumption and in turn reduce the incidence significantly. Ventilation of dwellings in regions where radon gas levels are high and avoidance of industrial carcinogens will also contribute to a reduction in lung cancer incidence.

Rare tumours

Giant cell carcinoma

This affects the younger age group more than other cancers, arises peripherally and is characterized histologically by multinucleate giant cells. The prognosis is poor.

Bronchoalveolar carcinoma

This arises more often in women with a peak incidence of 40–50 years. The cell of origin is the type 2 pneumocyte of the alveoli. It arises peripherally and the expectoration of large quantities of mucus is characteristic.

Clear cell carcinoma

This must be distinguished from a metastasis from a primary renal carcinoma which is the more common diagnosis.

Carcinoid

Bronchial carcinoids are the most common benign tumours, arising in the major bronchi. They are more common in the right lung and usually metabolically inactive but may produce carcinoid syndrome without liver metastases. They may occasionally be the site of ectopic ACTH production.

Future prospects

Current research is being directed towards chemotherapy dose intensification for SCLC with the haematological support of haemopoietic growth factors or bone marrow transplantation. The specific cytogenetic abnormalities seen in SCLC lend themselves to further study with a view to understanding the molecular biology of the disease.

8

Breast cancer

Epidemiology

There are 27 000 new cases of breast cancer and 15 000 deaths registered in the UK per annum. It is the most common malignancy in females, the average woman having a 1 in 12 chance of developing the disease at some point during her lifetime. The peak incidence is 50–70 years and only 0.5–1 per cent of cases will arise in men. It is a disease of the Western world being much less prevalent in the Far East, particularly Japan. There is an increased incidence in higher socio-economic groups.

Aetiology

Breast cancer risk is significantly increased when first degree relatives (e.g. sisters, aunts, mothers) have previously been affected, particularly if they develop cancer at an early stage or it is bilateral. A proportion of such cases has been found to have an abnormal gene located on chromosome 17. Familial cases may also have an increased risk of developing carcinoma of the ovary, endometrium, colon and rectum.

It is more common in women with an early menarche or a late menopause. An artificial menopause (surgical oophorectomy or radiation ovarian ablation) before the age of 35 years, increasing parity, young age (< 30 years) at first pregnancy and breast feeding are protective.

Japanese women have a low risk of developing breast cancer. Japanese migrants to the US eventually acquire the risk of the indigenous population, suggesting that there is an unknown environmental cofactor involved.

An increased incidence of breast cancer has been reported in atomic bomb survivors, women treated with radiotherapy for postpartum mastitis and women who underwent regular chest fluoroscopies to monitor the progress of iatrogenic pneumothorax as treatment for tuberculosis.

Bittner demonstrated that a virus transmitted via breast milk in mice led to the development of mammary tumours. A viral cause has not been demonstrated in humans with breast cancer.

Common benign lumps such as fibroadenomata do not progress to carcinoma, but atypical ductal hyperplasia on biopsy confers an increased risk of breast cancer.

Pathology

Variants worthy of special mention include:

1. Ductal carcinoma *in situ* (DCIS) – this is more common than lobular carcinoma *in situ* with a peak incidence 5–10 years later. Seventy to eighty per cent are symptomatic with a lump palpable in 60 per cent. Ten per cent present with nipple discharge, usually blood stained. Central necrosis leads to calcium deposition and therefore 50 per cent can be detected by mammography. Two per cent of surgically staged patients have spread to the axilla due to areas of unrecognized invasive carcinoma, and 40 per cent will progress to invasive carcinoma after biopsy alone.
2. Lobular carcinoma *in situ* (LCIS) – 70 per cent of cases arise in pre-menopausal women. It is usually undetectable clinically and cannot be seen on a mammogram. The rate of progression to carcinoma after biopsy alone is approximately 1 per cent per annum.
3. Inflammatory carcinoma – comprises only 2 per cent of all cases of breast cancer. Clinically there is ill-defined erythema, tenderness, induration, and eczema-like skin changes. It may be misdiagnosed as a breast abscess. Microscopically there is invasion of dermal lymphatics by tumour cells.
4. Paget's disease of the breast – a pre-malignant condition affecting the nipple and areola. Clinically there is erythema, dryness and fissuring of the nipple resembling eczema. Microscopically characterized by large, pale Paget cells within the epidermis which do not invade the dermis. Half have an associated lump, more than 90 per cent of which are invasive carcinomas. If no lump is palpable, 30 per cent will have an underlying invasive carcinoma and 70 per cent ductal carcinoma *in situ*.
5. Bilateral breast cancer – more common in those with a strong family history of breast cancer and those diagnosed at an early age. Synchronous primaries (i.e. two tumours occurring simultaneously) are rare occurring in less than 1 per cent of cases, while a metachronous primary (i.e. diagnosed 6 months or more after the original tumour) has an incidence of 1–2 per cent per year on follow-up. A second primary tumour is suggested by its being of a different histological type and differentiation to the original tumour with surrounding *in situ* changes.

Macroscopically, most carcinomas arise in the upper outer quadrant of the breast and are usually solitary although multifocal tumours may occur in the same or opposite breast. The tumour may be well circumscribed or diffusely infiltrating. The cut surface and texture will vary depending on the tumour type. For example, a schirrhous tumour will have a gritty texture and grey/white cut surface, while a colloid carcinoma will have a gelatinous texture.

Microscopically, breast cancers may be classified as 'lobular' arising in the lobules at the termination of the duct system of the breast or 'ductal' which arise from the ducts themselves. *In situ* carcinoma is diagnosed when all the malignant cells are confined to the lumen of the duct or lobule and do not breach the basement membrane. This contrasts with invasive carcinoma where malignant cells breach the basement membrane. The vast majority are ductal carcinomas but there are a number of variants including papillary, schirrhous, colloid, medullary and comedo carcinomas. Oestrogen and progesterone receptors are detectable, reaching high levels in well-differentiated tumours.

Natural history

The primary tumour enlarges and invades adjacent breast tissue, eventually leading to fixation to the pectoral fascia, serratus anterior muscle and ribs. The parietal pleura may be breached in neglected cases leading to transcoelomic spread within the pleural cavity. The dermal lymphatics may be invaded leading to 'peau d'orange' or satellite lesions. The dermis and epidermis may become infiltrated directly leading to nodules, plaques, ulceration or diffuse inflammatory changes. In neglected cases, the whole breast may be lost secondary to tumour necrosis (Fig. 8.1).

The likelihood of lymphatic involvement increases with increasing tumour size and decreasing tumour differentiation. Approximately one-third will have macroscopic or microscopic spread to the axillary nodes at the time of diagnosis. Involvement of the supraclavicular nodes is of particularly poor prognostic significance and is classified as a distant metastasis in the TNM staging. Medial tumours may involve the internal mammary nodes in the parasternal region.

The most common sites for distant metastases include bone, liver, lung, brain and skin. Breast cancer occasionally spreads to both ovaries, giving rise to 'Krukenberg tumours'. This phenomenon is also seen in stomach cancer.

Fig. 8.1 Neglected carcinoma of the breast. The breast has been destroyed over a period of many months.

Symptoms

The majority present with a breast lump, usually painless, which may be associated with a blood-stained nipple discharge, although patients detected by screening are likely to be asymptomatic. Less frequently the presentation is with lymphadenopathy or symptoms from metastases.

Signs

The lump is usually non-tender, well defined and most likely to be located in the upper outer quadrant. The overlying skin may be dimpled or frankly invaded by tumour leading to reddening, induration and nodular irregularity. Fixation to the skin or chest wall will limit mobility of the lump, and this should be sought by the clinician during physical examination. A very large lump will lead to obvious asymmetry of the breasts. There may be enlargement of the ipsilateral axillary lymph nodes, the mobility of which should be assessed as part of the clinical staging, and/or enlargement of the supraclavicular lymph nodes. Hepatomegaly may suggest metastatic infiltration while intrathoracic signs of collapse, consolidation or pleural effusion may suggest pulmonary or pleural metastases. Bone metastases are most frequent in the thoracic and lumbar spine and may lead to tenderness when pressure is applied to the affected vertebrae.

Differential diagnosis

A number of benign breast lumps may be clinically indistinguishable from carcinoma including fibroadenoma, breast abscess, fat necrosis, haematoma and galactocoele.

Rarer malignant tumours of the breast may occasionally cause confusion (see Rare tumours for more detailed description).

Investigations

Mammography

This comprises radiographs of the breasts using low energy X-rays to allow definition of the soft tissue detail and breast architecture. It may substantiate the clinical diagnosis of carcinoma, detect ductal carcinoma *in situ* in both the affected and contralateral breast, and localize the tumour to assist the planning of a biopsy or definitive surgical procedure. Carcinoma is suggested by an irregular mass lesion containing areas of microcalcification.

Breast ultrasound

This enables the radiologist to determine whether a lump is solid or cystic, the former being more likely to be malignant, and facilitates fine needle aspiration or needle biopsy of small lumps under direct vision, reducing the risk of a geographical miss and thereby increasing the sensitivity of the procedure.

Fine needle aspiration (FNA) cytology

This is a rapid, safe, relatively non-traumatic procedure which can be performed at an outpatient consultation and can provide a tissue diagnosis within hours. It should be performed whenever a palpable lump or suspicious area of induration is found, and is applicable to the primary tumour, regional lymph nodes or suspicious skin lesions.

Needle biopsy

This is performed under local anaesthetic and is a little more traumatic than FNA but gives a larger specimen of tissue for histological analysis.

Excision biopsy

An excision biopsy is mandatory when it is not possible to obtain a tissue diagnosis by FNA. The procedure is usually performed under general anaesthetic and the specimen can be sent for instant frozen section so that if a more radical operation is deemed necessary it can be performed immediately.

Exclusion of metastatic disease

The results of these investigations may influence the treatment planned, offer useful prognostic information and provide a valuable baseline assessment which may be of assistance in the future care of the patient:

1. Alkaline phosphatase, gammaglutamyltransferase to screen for liver metastases. A full blood count is also useful as a baseline measurement.
2. Chest X-ray to exclude lung metastases.

There is little evidence that routinely performing isotope bone scans to exclude skeletal metastases and liver ultrasounds to exclude liver metastases in asymptomatic patients is either clinically useful or cost effective, but they should be performed if there is any clinical suspicion of metastases at these sites. Suspicious areas on bone scan should be assessed further by plain radiographs, particularly if in weight-bearing bones.

Staging

The TNM staging is the most frequently used and can be used as a guide to management and prognosis:

T0   – No evidence of primary tumour.
TX   – Primary tumour cannot be assessed.
Tis   – Carcinoma *in situ*.
T1   – 2 cm or less in greatest dimension.
  1a   – 0.5 cm or less in greatest dimension.
  1b   – > 0.5 cm but not > 1 cm in greatest dimension.
  1c   – > 1 cm but not > 2 cm in greatest dimension.

T2	– > 2 cm but not > 5 cm in greatest dimension.
T3	– > 5 cm in greatest dimension.
T4	– Tumour of any size with extension to chest wall and/or skin.
4a	– Invasion of chest wall.
4b	– Oedema/peau d'orange, ulceration, satellite nodules confined to same breast.
4c	– Both 4a and 4b.
4d	– Inflammatory carcinoma.
N0	– No lymphadenopathy.
N1	– Ipsilateral mobile axillary nodes.
N2	– Ipsilateral axillary nodes fixed to one another or to adjacent structures.
N3	– Ipsilateral internal mammary node metastases.
M1	– Involvement of supraclavicular nodes or distant metastases.

Treatment

The aims of treatment are:

1. Locoregional control with optimal cosmesis.
2. Limitation of risk of developing distant metastatic disease and control of occult micrometastatic disease.
3. Minimization of short- and long-term treatment-related morbidity.

The treatment of breast cancer for an individual depends on the clinical stage of the disease, menopausal state and performance status of the patient. Ideally, the patient should be assessed in a combined breast clinic by both the surgeon and the clinical oncologist prior to any definitive treatment so that the optimum treatment can be instituted at the outset.

Treatment of local disease

Surgery

Surgery facilitates total clearance of the primary tumour and pathological examination of the primary tumour and regional lymph nodes. The operation used will depend on the size of the lump, its location within the breast, the size of the breast, the presence of multifocal disease or extensive carcinoma *in situ* in the surrounding breast tissue, and the surgeon's own practice and prejudices. Options for treating the primary tumour include:

1. Lumpectomy/wide local excision – the tumour is excised with a 2 cm margin of apparently uninvolved surrounding breast tissue. This gives an excellent cosmetic result (Fig. 8.2) as it preserves the breast bulk, even in women with small breasts. It is unsuitable for very large tumours (> 5 cm in maximum dimension), particularly if located centrally, or diffusely infiltrating carcinomas, particularly inflammatory carcinomas. Surrounding *in situ* disease will be left behind. Even if the excision margins are clear after microscopic examination of the specimen, there is a risk of local recurrence in the order of 20–30 per

cent without further local treatment.

2. Simple mastectomy – this involves complete removal of the involved breast. The pectoral muscles are preserved. Although a prosthesis will be required, the physical appearance of the chest wall will be far superior to that after a more radical mastectomy.
3. Modified radical (Patey) mastectomy – this constitutes a simple mastectomy but with removal of the pectoralis major and axillary lymph node dissection. There is thus added concave deformity of the chest wall compared with a simple mastectomy, but less deformity and better shoulder mobility than after a radical mastectomy.
4. Radical (Halstead) mastectomy – this operation involves en bloc

Fig. 8.2 Patient with a carcinoma of the left breast treated by lumpectomy and breast radiotherapy immediately after surgery (top) and 5 years after radiotherapy (bottom) (Courtesy of Dr J. Yarnold).

removal of the breast, pectoralis major and minor muscles, and the axillary contents. The cosmetic result is poor but the local control rate is as high as conservative surgery and post-operative radiotherapy.

In recent decades, there has been an increasing trend towards a philosophy of breast conservation which has been attributable to an improvement in the techniques of post-operative radiotherapy and an appreciation of its complementary role in the management of breast cancer. For a tumour 4 cm or less in maximum dimension, there is strong evidence that complete excision by lumpectomy combined with post-operative radiotherapy is as effective in obtaining local control as mastectomy alone, with 5 year disease-free survival rates of about 80 per cent. For tumours greater than 4 cm in maximum dimension, lumpectomy may still be performed and followed by radiotherapy. Due to this uncertainty and the poorer cosmetic result when a large tumour is treated conservatively, many surgeons will perform mastectomy for these larger tumours to maximize the chance of local control. Mastectomy is still the treatment of choice in certain situations:

1. When the patient wishes to have the breast removed.
2. Extensive ductal carcinoma *in situ*.
3. Paget's disease of the nipple.
4. Multifocal primaries.
5. Inflammatory carcinoma.
6. Treatment of malignant phylloides tumour or sarcoma.
7. A very large tumour in a small breast, particularly if centrally located.
8. Salvage treatment after failure of conservative therapy.
9. As a toilet procedure for a fungating tumour.

The psychosexual trauma and disturbance of body image that breast surgery can inflict should be considered. Patients for whom a mastectomy is planned should have the opportunity to see a trained breast care nurse counsellor prior to their surgery so that the implications of the operation can be sympathetically and skilfully discussed. Patients may wish to be fitted with a prosthesis to maintain their chest contour or undergo subsequent surgical reconstruction of the breast. Patients undergoing conservative treatment should also be offered counselling as studies suggest these patients experience psychological trauma similar to that of mastectomy patients.

The axilla is frequently a site for lymph node metastases, which in many cases cannot be detected clinically. The presence of lymph node metastases is a valuable prognostic factor, and correlates with the risk of the patient subsequently developing distant metastases. A surgical procedure to obtain lymph nodes for pathological analysis is therefore important in determining the need for adjuvant systemic therapy. In pre-menopausal women an axillary procedure should be performed in all cases as the results will determine the need for adjuvant chemotherapy. In post-menopausal women this is not essential as all patients receive adjuvant tamoxifen irrespective of node status (see later). There are two possible procedures:

1.   Axillary sampling – This entails removal of the lower lymph node group up to the level of the lower border of the pectoralis minor muscle. At least four nodes should be obtained for histological examination. If these nodes are not involved by cancer, it is unlikely that nodes higher in the axilla will be either.
2.   Axillary dissection – This is a more extensive surgical procedure comprising removal of the axillary contents up to the level of the axillary vein. Twenty to thirty nodes may be retrieved for the pathologist, giving more detailed prognostic information. It also has the advantage of being a therapeutic manoeuvre in its own right, lessening the risk of axillary recurrence. It has the disadvantage of increasing the surgical morbidity, resulting in local sensory loss, stiffness of the shoulder and risk of lymphoedema of the ipsilateral arm.

Radiotherapy

Radiotherapy is indicated in all patients treated by lumpectomy or wide local excision, in order to give local control equivalent to mastectomy (5–10 per cent 5 year local relapse rate). After simple mastectomy, radiotherapy reduces the risk of chest wall recurrence threefold from 30 per cent at 5 years to 10 per cent, equivalent to that after radical mastectomy. There is no proven survival advantage for immediate radiotherapy v. radiotherapy deferred until relapse. Some patient selection after mastectomy is necessary, and so radiotherapy is offered to those at particularly high risk of chest wall relapse such as tumours that have not been completely excised at a microscopic level, tumours with positive axillary lymph nodes or poorly differentiated tumours. External beam radiotherapy is administered to the breast alone. Radiotherapy to the breast may also be given by the implantation of radioactive sources – usually wires of Iridium[192] which has the advantage of delivering a very high dose of radiation to a localized volume of tissue with a good cosmetic result. It is used either to boost the tumour bed after external beam irradiation of the breast or as a treatment of scar relapse after previous radiotherapy.

External beam radiotherapy may also be given to the axilla if the axillary node status is not known or axillary node sampling is positive. Radiotherapy to the axilla does prevent relapse but again is not proven to enhance survival when used early as opposed to when it is used as a salvage treatment at time of axillary relapse. It should not be given routinely after axillary dissection irrespective of node status as there will be a considerable risk of lymphoedema of the arm and stiffness of the shoulder which in some cases will be incapacitating.

Chemotherapy/hormone manipulation

Inoperable tumours are initially treated with systemic therapy – chemotherapy for pre-menopausal women and hormone therapy for post-menopausal women, as a high proportion of such patients will have occult metastatic disease. Once maximal response to systemic therapy has been attained, if there is no evidence of metastatic disease, the breast may be treated by surgery with or without radiotherapy.

Adjuvant systemic therapy

Adjuvant systemic therapy complements the role of radiotherapy or surgery to the breast. The former acts upon cancer cells which have already metastasized outside the breast and its regional lymphatics while the latter reduces the local relapse rate. It is now widely accepted that adjuvant systemic therapy is of proven benefit in reducing the risk of distant relapse due to metastatic spread, and that this translates into a significant benefit in disease-free and overall survival. Breast cancer is statistically an important cancer accounting for much morbidity and mortality among women, and so only a small increase in these parameters will be worthwhile. There are two main types of adjuvant systemic therapy.

Hormone manipulation

Tamoxifen is an antioestrogen which acts by blocking the action of oestradiol on its receptors within the cytoplasm and nucleus of the tumour cells. The dose is 20 mg once daily. There is no evidence that a higher dose is any more effective. It has been proven to be an effective adjuvant agent in women over 50 years (i.e. predominantly post-menopausal), particularly those who are axillary lymph node positive, prolonging disease-free and overall survival by 20–30 per cent. Recent evidence suggests that it is also effective in women under 50 years (i.e. predominantly pre-menopausal) but to a lesser degree than in post-menopausal women. The greatest benefit is seen in node positive women particularly if the primary expresses high levels of the oestrogen receptor. There is also evidence that tamoxifen decreases the risk of developing a contralateral primary breast cancer. Side effects are rarely severe enough to warrant discontinuation of tamoxifen. The most common complaint is that of sweating and flushing. The cost of such prolonged drug treatment is considerable – estimates in 1990 indicated that the cost per life saved is £19 000 for node negative women and £5000 for node positive women, rising to £47 500 for node negative women if tamoxifen is given for 5 years.

Radiation-induced menopause is only indicated for pre-menopausal women, producing improvements in disease-free and overall survival of 20–30 per cent. External beam irradiation is administered to the lower pelvis as 4–5 daily fractions and its effect on the ovary is irreversible.

Surgical oophorectomy is an alternative to radiation-induced menopause and entails removal of both ovaries. It is only indicated in pre-menopausal women. It is as effective as radiation-induced menopause but has the advantage of not relying on patient compliance and is in the long term more cost effective than tamoxifen.

Gonadotrophin-releasing hormone analogues act by leading to hormonal down-regulation of the hypothalamo–pituitary axis, resulting in a complete cessation of ovarian oestrogen production. Either Goserelin or Leuprolide is suitable but they are expensive. They are given once monthly as a subcutaneous injection and their effect is reversible.

Chemotherapy

Adjuvant chemotherapy is of greatest benefit in the management of axillary lymph node positive pre-menopausal women. Chemotherapy produces a 28 per cent reduction in the annual odds of recurrence and 17 per cent reduction in the annual odds of dying, the effect persisting for at least 10 years. There is a beneficial effect in post-menopausal women of about half this order of magnitude, but chemotherapy is not routinely used in this group due to the greater effectiveness and more favourable toxicity profile of tamoxifen. The role of chemotherapy in node negative pre-menopausal women is yet to be defined. There is evidence that 6 months of combination chemotherapy using at least three drugs is optimal and the most tried and tested regime is CMF comprising:

- Cyclophosphamide 100 mg/m² po day 1 to day 14.
- Methotrexate 40 mg/m² iv day 1 and day 8.
- 5-fluorouracil 600 mg/m² iv day 1 and day 8.
- Repeat cycle 4 weekly for 6 cycles.

There is evidence that the benefit of adjuvant chemotherapy may be additive to that of radiation menopause in pre-menopausal women and tamoxifen in post-menopausal women, but combined treatment is not routine practice in this country.

Treatment of metastatic disease

The disease is incurable at this stage, and treatment is aimed to palliate symptoms and maintain the patient as active as possible with as few side effects as possible and the least inconvenience.

Surgery

There is no role for breast surgery in the patient with metastatic disease provided a tissue diagnosis has already been obtained and satisfactory local control of the breast tumour can be achieved by other treatment modalities. Pleurodesis is sometimes of value in the treatment of recurrent malignant pleural effusions, and internal fixation is indicated if fracture of a weight-bearing bone has occurred or is imminent.

Radiotherapy

The natural history of breast cancer dictates that most patients with metastatic breast cancer will have symptomatic bone metastases leading up to the terminal phase of the disease, although some will also be troubled by brain, cutaneous or choroidal metastases. Radiotherapy is the treatment of choice for metastases causing local symptoms.

Hormone therapy

Tamoxifen is the agent of first choice in post-menopausal women who are not taking it as adjuvant therapy, producing an objective response in 40 per cent of oestrogen receptor positive tumours and 10 per cent of oestrogen negative ones. Response rate is greatest in those with high levels of oestrogen receptor, usually those with well-differentiated tumours and the elderly. Median duration of response is 10 months. Medroxyprogesterone acetate (200–400 mg bd) or megestrol acetate (80 mg bd) produce a further objective response in about 10 per cent of those progressing on tamoxifen, particularly if there has been a previous hormone response. Once second line hormone therapy has failed, a further hormone response to other agents such as the adrenal antagonist aminoglutethimide and the anabolic steroid nandrolone is very unlikely. Unless already performed as adjuvant therapy, pre-menopausal women with metastatic disease should undergo some form of artificial menopause with the expectation of a 30 per cent objective response. Tamoxifen also has a worthwhile effect if there is further disease progression.

Chemotherapy

There is no strong evidence that the use of chemotherapy for the treatment of metastatic disease prolongs survival, and indeed its toxicity may be detrimental to the patient's quality of life. Many would therefore argue that it should be instituted only for the control of symptoms or rapidly progressive disease in good performance status patients. Chemotherapy is effective against soft tissue metastases but is less effective than radiotherapy for palliating bone metastases. CMF is again the most frequently used, producing objective responses of 50–60 per cent and a median duration of response of 7 months. At least 6 cycles are administered unless chemoresistence is demonstrated by progression during treatment. After 6 cycles the treatment is continued for as long as some objective response is obtained unless toxicity is so severe as to compromise the patient's quality of life and warrant termination of treatment. Those patients failing CMF can be treated with an adriamycin-containing regimen with the expectation of a few further responders.

Tumour-related complications

Hypercalcaemia, spinal cord compression and pathological fracture are seen in patients with widespread skeletal metastases (see Chapter 22). Disseminated intravascular coagulation is seen in advanced disease when the tumour burden is high and usually heralds the terminal phase of the disease. Mucin production by the tumour may activate the clotting cascade causing uncontrolled coagulation coupled with a physiological thrombolysis leading to occlusion of both small and large blood vessels. Consumption of clotting factors deranges thrombin time and activated partial thromboplastin time resulting in a bleeding tendency, while platelet consumption leads to thrombocytopaenia manifested as epistaxis, petechiae and bruising. Fibrin degradation products are elevated.

Treatment-related complications

Radiotherapy

During treatment the patient may experience breast erythema, swelling, skin irritation and tenderness which settle within 2–4 weeks of completing treatment. Late complications of radiotherapy occur in less than 5 per cent and include cutaneous necrosis, telangiectasia, rib fractures, radionecrosis of ribs, radiation costochondritis and pneumonitis. A slightly increased risk of death from cardiovascular disease has been reported. Axillary irradiation is associated with late morbidity such as lymphoedema of the arm, stiffness of the shoulder, radiation injury to the brachial plexus and radionecrosis of the proximal humerus, although with current techniques the incidence is less than 5 per cent if radiotherapy is not combined with surgery.

Chemotherapy

A recall of the radiation skin reaction may occur with adriamycin-containing regimens. Adverse effects are otherwise not specific for breast cancer (see Chapter 6).

Hormone therapy

Tamoxifen may cause a 'flare' in bone pain when prescribed for skeletal metastases and acute hypercalcaemia is recognized. It should be noted that tamoxifen can significantly potentiate the anticoagulant effect of warfarin.

Prognosis

In operable cases, the 5 and 10 year survivals are approximately 80 per cent and 60 per cent for node negative patients and 60 per cent and 40 per cent for node positive patients respectively. Poor prognostic factors include:

1.   Tumour stage:

- Increasing size of primary tumour.
- Local invasion to involve chest wall or skin.
- Involvement of the axillary nodes or distant metastases.
- Inflammatory carcinoma.

2.   Microscopic features:

- Invasive v. non-invasive tumours.
- Poorly differentiated tumours.
- Lymphatic vessel invasion.
- Vascular invasion.

3. Oestrogen and progesterone receptor negative tumours.

4. Markers of rapid cell proliferation:

- High thymidine labelling index.
- High S-phase fraction.

5. Cathepsin D over expression.

6. Positivity for the oncogene C-*erb*B-2.

Screening

Screening should permit the diagnosis of a higher proportion of early stages of the disease. As early stage at diagnosis is an important favourable prognostic factor, this should translate into a reduction in mortality from breast cancer. About 20 per cent of screen detected cancers will be *in situ*, a further 20 per cent will be invasive cancers less than 1 cm in diameter and a similar percentage 1–2 cm.

Breast self-examination (BSE) should be routinely practised by women at the same time each month to take account of the variation in breast size and consistency with the menstrual cycle. However, to date BSE has not conclusively been shown to have decreased breast cancer mortality and there has been concern as to the stress of such a practise. 'Breast awareness' has been proposed whereby a woman has an appreciation of her breasts and reports any untoward findings to her doctor for immediate assessment.

Mammography is a sensitive means of detecting carcinomas, often before the lump is palpable by the patient or clinician, thereby facilitating the detection of early breast cancers with a particularly good prognosis. There is currently a National Breast Screening Programme in operation, with all women aged 50–64 being offered 3 yearly single oblique view mammograms. Women 65 years or more will be screened on request. It is estimated that such a program will result in a mortality reduction of 20–30 per cent. There is at present no consensus as to whether pre-menopausal women should be included in such a screening programme, although women with a family history of breast cancer should be offered regular screening.

Prevention

Breast cancer is sufficiently common to make prevention a worthwhile exercise. Patient education is necessary, with emphasis on those individuals at particular risk of breast cancer, e.g. those with a family history of breast cancer. Any method of prevention must be easy to comply with, free of short- and long-term adverse effects and not consume too many healthcare resources. The difference in dietary fat intake between the Western world and Africa and Asia contributes to the geographical variation in incidence. A reduction in the proportion of daily calories obtained from dietary fat could make a significant impact on the incidence of breast cancer. It has been estimated that a decrease in dietary fat from the average of 40 per cent to 20 per cent would decrease the incidence of breast cancer several fold. Dietary manipulation has the advantage of being inherently cost effective, and may reduce morbidity and mortality from cardiovascular and cerebrovascular disease and colorectal cancer. Uncertainty exists as to when such a dietary adjustment should be instituted and for how long, although its other advantages make it desirable to make it a lifelong commitment.

Breast cancer is the only malignant disease for which large scale trials are in progress to determine whether chemoprevention is feasible but is only in the early stages of clinical testing. Tamoxifen 20 mg daily is currently being evaluated in several large placebo-controlled trials. There are no data available to confirm its efficacy in chemoprevention, but toxicity studies have suggested that it may reduce cholesterol and thereby indirectly have additional health benefits. The progesterone drug Gestodene is a strong candidate as a chemoprevention agent as it can be conveniently incorporated into an oral contraceptive preparation for widespread, long-term use.

Rare tumours

Cystosarcoma phylloides

This is much less common than carcinoma and arises in elderly women. It is usually a large tumour and well circumscribed, often indistinguishable from a fibroadenoma or carcinoma. Most behave in an indolent manner with slowly progressive local infiltration of the breast with only a few metastasizing to distant sites. Treatment is by simple mastectomy and axillary lymph node sampling or dissection is not indicated. There is no role for radiotherapy or systemic adjuvant therapy post-operatively.

Lymphoma

This has a peak incidence of 50–55 years and is usually a diffuse high grade non-Hodgkin's lymphoma. Staging and treatment is as for any other extranodal lymphoma and mastectomy is not indicated.

Liposarcoma

This is a very rare tumour which may arise from a phylloides tumour or a fibroadenoma and has a peak incidence of 50 years. Lymphatic involvement is not seen and about one-quarter will develop distant metastases.

Leiomyosarcoma

This, like liposarcoma, has a peak incidence at about 50 years but 25 per cent arise in men. There is a low incidence of metastatic disease.

Osteosarcoma

The breast is a rare extraosseous site for this tumour with a peak incidence of 60–65 years. One-third will recur locally after radical surgery and 70–80 per cent will develop distant metastases.

Future prospects

Effective chemoprevention remains a possible way to decrease the incidence of breast cancer, particularly in those individuals perceived to be at high risk of developing the disease. The management of breast cancer will be improved by prospectively randomized, controlled trials addressing the issue of adjuvant therapy in the node negative pre-menopausal woman, and the synergistic effect of chemotherapy with artificial menopause or tamoxifen in the relevant age groups. The optimum management of screen-detected ductal and lobular carcinoma *in situ* also remains uncertain and is the subject of intense study.

9
Gastrointestinal cancer

Carcinoma of the oesophagus

Epidemiology

There are 5000 new cases of oesophageal cancer and approximately the same number of deaths registered in the UK per annum. Overall there is a male to female ratio of 3:2 although tumours of the upper third are more common in females, and the peak incidence is 60–70 years. The highest incidence is found in China, Iran and Transkei.

Aetiology

Tobacco smoking is a strong risk factor for oesophageal cancer.

The regular consumption of alcoholic spirits predisposes to cancer due to a chronic irritative effect on the mucosa. Carcinogenic contaminants of alcoholic drinks have also been implicated in some cases, e.g. the home-made beer consumed by the Xhosa people in Transkei.

Barrett's oesophagus is characterized by glandular metaplasia of the squamous epithelium of the lower third of the oesophagus, usually in response to chronic gastro-oesophageal reflux from a hiatus hernia. Patients are at risk of developing an adenocarcinoma of the oesophagus.

In achalasia there is chronic stasis and pooling of food and secretions in a dilated oesophagus due to a loss of oesophageal motility. The increased risk of cancer is due to prolonged contact of the mucosa with carcinogens within the food or produced from food by the action of bacteria.

Patterson–Brown–Kelly syndrome (Plummer–Vinson syndrome) is characterized by koilionychia, iron deficiency anaemia, the presence of an 'oesophageal web' in the upper third of the oesophagus on barium swallow and is usually seen in women. It leads to a carcinoma of the upper third of the oesophagus in the post-cricoid region.

Tylosis is a rare, dominantly inherited condition characterized by palmar and plantar hyperkeratosis and a strong predisposition to oesophageal cancer.

Pathology

Approximately 40–50 per cent arise in the middle third of the oesophagus, 40–50 per cent in the lower third, and less than 10 per cent in the upper third, the tumour appearing nodular, ulcerating or diffusely infiltrative. If there is oesophageal obstruction, the proximal oesophagus is frequently dilated and contains food debris. A fistula may occasionally exist between the oesophagus and trachea or bronchial tree, and there may be evidence of an aspiration pneumonia particularly in the lower lobes of the lungs.

Cancers of the upper two-thirds of the oesophagus are invariably squamous cell carcinomas. Those in the lower third are most commonly squamous but one-third are adenocarcinomas which may have arisen in an area of metaplasia such as Barrett's oesophagus. These must be distinguished from adenocarcinoma of the proximal stomach which has infiltrated the oesophagus. Insidious spread along the submucosa is common and may lead to skip lesions some distance from the main tumour.

Natural history

The tumour will spread within the oesophagus both longitudinally and circumferentially, eventually resulting in complete oesophageal obstruction. Invasion through the deeper layers of the oesophageal wall will result in spread to the surrounding mediastinal structures such as the trachea, main brochi (especially left), pleura, lung, vertebrae and great vessels.

The pattern of lymphatic involvement reflects the complex blood supply to the oesophagus. Tumours of the upper third will spread to the deep cervical and supraclavicular nodes, those of the middle third to the mediastinal, paratracheal and subcarinal nodes, and those of the lower third to the nodes of the coeliac axis below the diaphragm.

The venous drainage of parts of the oesophagus is into the portal circulation and so the liver is the most common site of distant metastases, although the lungs and skeleton may also be involved.

Symptoms

Dysphagia is the most common presenting symptom. A middle aged or elderly patient complaining of this symptom should be considered to have oesophageal cancer until proven otherwise and referral to a gastroenterologist is mandatory. The symptom begins insidiously as a sensation of food sticking, usually when solids such as meat have been eaten, progresses so that there is difficulty with softer foods/liquids and may be associated with retrosternal discomfort due to stretching of the oesophagus and increased peristalsis.

Regurgitation usually accompanies severe dysphagia. Retrosternal discomfort is followed by effortless regurgitation of the oesophageal contents. These do not taste sour as they have not entered the stomach. This contrasts with gastro-oesophageal reflux where there will be a strong taste of acid.

Weight loss is due to both reduced calorie intake due to dysphagia and/or regurgitation, and the non-specific effects of malignancy.

Recurrent aspiration is a problem in patients with proximal tumours leading to overspill into the upper respiratory tract or with a fistula connecting the oesophagus to the lower respiratory tract. The patient experiences a severe bout of coughing within a short time of swallowing, and may expectorate solid material from the food bolus. Both predispose to recurrent chest infections which may be fatal.

Signs

Women with Plummer–Vinson syndrome may appear anaemic and have koilionychia, while alcoholics may have stigmata of chronic liver disease. There is often evidence of malnutrition, the degree of which is dependent on the duration and severity of dysphagia and whether there has been a history of alcoholism. In cases of oesophageal obstruction the patient may even be dehydrated due to poor fluid intake. There is usually no palpable evidence of disease although an epigastric mass may be palpable in tumours of the lower third of the oesophagus and if there are large intra-abdominal lymph nodes. The cervical and supraclavicular lymph nodes should be palpated carefully. Hepatomegaly suggests metastatic disease but may indicate fatty infiltration in heavy drinkers.

Differential diagnosis

Care has to be taken not to confuse a tumour arising from the oesophageal mucosa with a tumour arising from an adjacent structure and invading into the oesophagus, e.g. carcinoma of the left main bronchus (most often squamous or small cell carcinoma), carcinoma of the fundus of the stomach or gastro-oesophageal junction (adenocarcinoma). Other differential diagnoses include a benign oesophageal stricture due to chronic gastro-oesophageal reflux, achalasia, and hysteria although this is only a diagnosis made after excluding all other possible causes.

Investigations

The oesophagus starts at the lower border of the cricoid cartilage at the level of the 6th cervical vertebra, approximately 15 cm from the incisor teeth. It is 25 cm in length, entering the stomach at the level of the 10th thoracic vertebra (i.e. approximately 40 cm from the incisors).

Serum alkaline phosphatase, gammaglutamyltransferase and a liver ultrasound should be performed in all cases to screen for liver metastases and a chest X-ray is performed to exclude lung metastases and mediastinal lymphadenopathy.

Barium swallow and meal

A barium swallow will outline the oesophageal lumen, a carcinoma appearing as a stricture, filling defect or abnormal flow of barium (Fig. 9.1). This investigation will not give a tissue diagnosis and all patients should proceed to endoscopy.

Endoscopy

This is the investigation of choice as it allows the tumour to be visualized directly and facilitates a biopsy for histology and brushings for cytology.

As with the barium meal, it allows a thorough evaluation of the stomach, which is particularly important in tumours of the lower third of the oesophagus, and is the most sensitive means of detecting small primary tumours and skip lesions.

CT scan of the thorax

This provides information on the local extent of the disease with respect to invasion beyond the oesophagus and is of value in planning radiotherapy or surgery because it will also allow an assessment of the regional lymph nodes, liver and lungs.

Staging

There is no formal staging system in routine clinical use.

Treatment

Many patients will be poorly nourished which lessens their tolerance of radical treatment and therefore referral to a dietitian is advisable in all cases. A liquidizer may help the patient to continue eating food prepared at home. It may be necessary for the patient to be given liquid dietary supplements to maintain calorie intake and nasogastric tube feeding may be the only means of maintaining nutrition.

Fig. 9.1 Barium swallow showing an irregular, malignant stricture of the middle third of the oesophagus. Note the small pool of barium at the top of the stricture.

Radical

Surgery

This is the treatment of choice for localized lower third tumours as:

1. This is the most surgically accessible part of oesophagus.
2. The anterior curvature of spinal cord makes radiotherapy planning more difficult.
3. High dose irradiation of the cardia of the stomach can result in a severe erosive gastritis.

Contraindications to surgery are:

1. Vocal cord palsy – this indicates infiltration of or pressure on the recurrent laryngeal nerve, suggesting spread beyond the oesophagus.
2. Invasion of great vessels (aorta, superior vena cava), pericardium.
3. Broncho-oesophageal fistula.
4. Cervical/coeliac node involvement clinically or radiologically.
5. Distant metastases.
6. Poor performance status, severe malnutrition.

Tumours of the middle third can be treated by an Ivor Lewis two-stage oesophagectomy. The stomach is mobilized via upper abdominal incision, the oesophagus approached via the right 5th intercostal space, the tumour is resected allowing a 5 cm margin of macroscopically normal oesophagus, and the oesophagus is then reanastomosed. The operative mortality is high at up to 20 per cent depending on patient selection and the surgeon's skill. For tumours of the lower third, a left thoracoabdominal incision is made, the tumour mobilized and resected with reanastomosis of the transected oesophagus.

Radiotherapy

Radiotherapy is the treatment of choice for tumours of the upper third, where surgery would be difficult, but can be used for tumours elsewhere that are not amenable to surgery. The treatment-related mortality is much lower than radical surgery. Although distant metastases are a contraindication to radical radiotherapy, extra-oesophageal invasion may still be encompassed within the radiation high dose zone. Treatment is given daily over 4 to 6 weeks. Pre-operative and post-operative radiotherapy does not prolong survival and has no clearly defined role in the management of this disease.

Palliative

Dysphagia and regurgitation are the symptoms most often requiring treatment. Both are extremely distressing and can erode the quality of life significantly.

Radiotherapy

A short course of radiotherapy will relieve dysphagia in most patients with acceptable short-term morbidity and can usually be repeated if necessary. This may be given as a course of external beam irradiation or intra-luminal irradiation whereby a high activity radiation source is inserted directly into the oesophagus via a nasogastric tube.

Other treatments

Fibre-optic endoscopy permits a number of procedures to be performed under direct vision. Dilatation using metal bougies allows a stricture to be stretched and relieves dysphagia to some degree in the majority, although the procedure may need to be repeated a number of times during the patient's remaining lifetime. Alternatively, an endoprosthesis such as an Atkinson tube may be inserted to maintain oesophageal patency and is particularly useful in relieving recurrent aspiration due to a fistula. Laser therapy may be given to coagulate a bleeding tumour or to unblock an obstructed oesophagus.

Tumour-related complications

Aspiration of food into the respiratory tract will lead to pneumonia which may be further complicated by lung abscess and empyema. Haemorrhage is a rare but potentially fatal local tumour complication.

Treatment-related complications

Surgery

Loss of oesophageal integrity after surgical resection may lead to a fistula or mediastinitis which may be fatal, while pneumothorax, pulmonary collapse and pneumonia may complicate a thoracotomy.

Radiotherapy

During treatment, it is inevitable that the patient will experience some worsening of dysphagia due to a radiation oesophagitis. This can be minimized by avoidance of very hot or cold food/fluids, and relieved by mucaine 10 ml tds sipped slowly. Anorexia and nausea/vomiting are likely if stomach and/or liver is included in the radiation fields and will be helped by a regular antiemetic. Radiation pneumonitis is uncommon and usually subclinical, although it may cause a dry cough, fever and dyspnoea. Oesophageal stricture may occur from 6 months after radiotherapy giving rise to dysphagia, and needs to be distinguished from recurrent tumour, preferably by endoscopy so that a dilatation can be performed simultaneously.

Prognosis

Five year survival is only 5–10 per cent and is usually due to many cases having occult lymph node or distant metastases at presentation.

Screening/prevention

Informing the public of the risks of tobacco and alcohol could reduce the incidence of oesophageal cancer. In areas of very high prevalence, screening is a beneficial and cost-effective exercise. In the UK, patients with a Barrett's oesophagus should be offered annual endoscopic examination due to their high risk of developing carcinoma.

Rare tumours

Adenoid cystic carcinoma

This is a tumour arising from the mucous glands of the mucosa and is of the same type as those arising in the parotid salivary gland and elsewhere.

Small cell carcinoma

Although infiltration from an underlying lung primary should be considered, a primary tumour of this type has been described.

Melanoma

This is a rare site for mucosal melanoma. Prognosis will be very poor due to advanced stage at presentation.

Carcinoid

This is an uncommon site for this rare tumour. It should be treated as elsewhere by surgical resection.

Leiomyosarcoma

This tumour arises from the smooth muscle fibres of the oesophageal wall. It is best treated by radical surgery combined with radiotherapy.

Carcinoma of the stomach

Epidemiology

There are 12 000 new cases and 11 000 deaths registered in the UK per annum with a peak incidence of 50–70 years and a male to female ratio of 2:1. Blood group O confers some protection against developing stomach cancer while blood group A is associated with a higher incidence of the diffuse form of stomach cancer. The incidence is very high in Japan and Chile, and increased in lower socio-economic groups.

Aetiology

The stomach is exposed to a variety of carcinogens both ingested and produced from the action of bacteria within the stomach. Nitrosamines have been implicated in stomach cancer, as has a diet rich in smoked foodstuffs.

Atrophic gastritis and achlorhydria both increase the risk of developing stomach cancer, in the case of pernicious anaemia by fivefold. This may be related to bacterial overgrowth and increased production of endogenous carcinogens. A partial gastrectomy or gastroenterostomy is also associated with an increased cancer risk, probably due to a chronic reflux of bile salts into the stomach. An adenoma–carcinoma sequence is recognized but is much rarer than in the large bowel.

There is an increased risk in those with a family history of diffuse stomach cancer and blood group A.

Pathology

Stomach cancers usually form discrete ulcerating lesions, but may be nodular or polypoid. They are occasionally diffusely infiltrating leading to obliteration of the stomach lumen. Fifty per cent arise in the pyloric region while of those arising in the body, most are found along the lesser curvature.

Ninety-five per cent are adenocarcinomas, and 5 per cent squamous carcinoma or adenoacanthoma (adenocarcinoma with areas of squamous metaplasia). There may be evidence of prior intestinal metaplasia and carcinoma *in situ* in the surrounding mucosa.

Natural history

Cancers spread longitudinally and circumferentially within the stomach, and as with carcinoma of the oesophagus insidious submucosal spread is frequent. Progressive invasion into the muscle layer of the stomach wall eventually leads to invasion of the serosa and in turn invasion of adjacent viscera such as the omentum, pancreas, spleen, left kidney and adrenal. Invasion superiorly by a tumour of the fundus may result in occlusion of the lower third of the oesophagus leading to dysphagia and regurgitation. There is a propensity for transcoelomic spread with diffuse peritoneal seeding leading to ascites and ovarian deposits (Krukenberg tumours), particularly with the 'signet ring' variant.

Spread to the regional lymph nodes (gastric, gastroduodenal, splenic and coeliac groups) occurs early in the natural history, and Virchow's node in the left supraclavicular fossa may be involved (Troisier's sign).

Distant spread occurs to the liver via the portal venous circulation, lung, bone, brain and skin.

Symptoms

The patient frequently presents with non-specific gastrointestinal symptoms such as epigastric discomfort, anorexia, nausea, vomiting and weight loss which are frequently confused with a benign condition such as peptic ulceration or gastritis, and may even be relieved by antacids or H2 antagonists.

Others present with the symptoms of an iron deficiency anaemia and stomach cancer should always be considered in the assessment of such patients.

A more acute presentation may occur with stomach perforation, haematemesis and/or melaena.

Signs

At presentation, many will have been losing weight, and cachexia is a frequent finding. An epigastric mass may be palpable and there may be palpable lymph nodes in the left supraclavicular fossa. The liver may be enlarged, tender and knobbly suggesting metastatic infiltration, and there may be ascites. Non-metastatic manifestations such as dermatomyositis and acanthosis nigricans may also be seen.

Differential diagnosis

This includes:

1.   Inflammatory conditions, e.g. peptic ulcer.
2.   Other malignant gastric tumours, e.g. lymphoma, leiomyosarcoma.
3.   Benign gastric tumours, e.g. leiomyoma, carcinoid.

Investigations

Barium meal

Double contrast barium meal will outline the gastric mucosa and is a sensitive investigation for detecting mucosal abnormalities. Although carcinomas often have a characteristic appearance, there may be confusion with benign peptic ulcers and therefore further investigation to obtain a tissue diagnosis is mandatory.

Fibre-optic endoscopy

This permits direct visualization of the gastric mucosa, allowing a more accurate assessment of the macroscopic appearances of an abnormality. It also permits biopsy and brushings for cytology to give a tissue diagnosis.

CT scan of the abdomen

This will provide the surgeon with information regarding invasion beyond the stomach and whether the regional lymph nodes are enlarged, and thereby help to determine whether the tumour is operable.

Tests to exclude metastatic disease

1.   Serum alkaline phosphatase and gammaglutamyltransferase as screening tests for liver metastases.
2.   Liver ultrasound to exclude metastases.
3.   Chest X-ray to exclude lung metastases.

4. Carcinoembryonic antigen – may be elevated reflecting tumour burden but is not routinely of value. It may permit early diagnosis of distant and/or local relapse after curative treatment.

Staging

There is no formal staging system in routine clinical use.

Treatment

Radical

Surgery

This is the only potentially curative treatment but only two-thirds of patients are deemed operable after full staging investigations and a further two-thirds of these will be found to be inoperable, meaning that overall only 1 in 6 patients stand any chance of being cured. A partial or total gastrectomy is mandatory in operable cases depending on the size and site of the tumour.

Radiotherapy

Radiotherapy has no curative role in treatment due to the dose limiting toxicity induced in the stomach and adjacent structures such as the small bowel and transverse colon when a high dose of radiation is administered. Adjuvant post-operative radiotherapy does not significantly improve survival and is not routinely practised – most patients will die of distant metastases rather than local recurrence.

Palliative

Surgery

Intestinal bypass surgery is effective in relieving gastric outflow obstruction while gastrectomy may be justified in the presence of metastatic disease when massive bleeding cannot be controlled by less invasive methods.

Radiotherapy

Radiotherapy is valuable in relieving the local symptoms of inoperable disease such as dysphagia, haemorrhage or pain due to retroperitoneal infiltration.

Chemotherapy

This may be of value in relieving symptoms from metastatic disease, particularly for lung and liver metastases. The most active single agent is 5-fluorouracil which may be used in combination with other drugs such as adriamycin and mitomycin C (FAM).

Endoscopic procedures

Laser therapy is particularly useful for the photocoagulation of a persistently bleeding tumour or debulking of a large tumour which is narrowing the oesophageal lumen. An oesophageal endoprosthesis is occasionally of benefit for a tumour of the upper stomach which is occluding the oesophagus from below.

Tumour-related complications

Haemorrhage may be life threatening if a major gastric vessel is eroded while chronic blood loss will lead to an iron deficiency anaemia with a reduced serum ferritin. Invasion through the stomach wall into the peritoneal cavity may lead to leakage of gastric contents and an acute peritonitis. Pyloric stenosis may lead to gastric outflow obstruction eventually leading to episodes of projectile vomiting, visible peristalsis, a 'succussion splash' and obstruction. Mucin secretion by the tumour may result in activation of the plasmin/plasminogen cascade leading to a disseminated intravascular coagulation manifested by abnormal clotting, thrombocytopaenia and raised fibrin degradation products (see Chapter 8).

Treatment-related complications

Surgery

Loss of stomach volume will lead to a feeling of fullness after small portions of food, while loss of gastric acidity may predispose to iron deficiency. Impaired intrinsic factor production will lead to vitamin B12 deficiency secondary to impaired absorption at the terminal ileum resulting in a macrocytic anaemia while impaired digestion may result in malabsorption and a 'dumping syndrome' due to hypoglycaemia. Stomal ulceration and ultimately a second malignancy may occur.

Radiotherapy

During treatment the patient will experience some degree of anorexia, nausea and vomiting. High doses of radiation to the stomach may result in a chronic gastritis. The left kidney may receive a dose sufficient to impair its function permanently which will be relevant if the right kidney function is subnormal. Radiation enteritis and colitis is also a recognized complication.

Prognosis

The median survival for patients with unresectable disease is about 4 months and the 5 year survival is less than 10 per cent overall rising to 15–20 per cent in those undergoing successful surgical resection. Early gastric cancer has a good 5 year survival of 70 per cent or more.

Screening/prevention

A screening programme of double contrast barium examination of the stomach and gastroscopy has been successfully implemented in Japan. This has lead to a greater proportion of early cancers being detected, resulting in a decline in mortality. Gastric juice analysis suggests that a low pepsinogen 1 and high gastrin are good predictors for gastritis and cancer risk.

Rare tumours

Leiomyoma

This is a benign tumour arising from smooth muscle of the stomach wall, often found incidentally during investigation of the upper gastrointestinal tract but they may ulcerate leading to haematemesis.

Carcinoid

The stomach is a very uncommon site for carcinoid tumours which are best treated surgically (see Chapter 14).

Lymphoma

The stomach is a common site for extranodal lymphoma which is usually a high grade diffuse non-Hodgkin's lymphoma. Perforation is a risk if the initial management is not surgical due to the tumour's great radiosensitivity and chemosensitivity.

Carcinoma of the pancreas

Epidemiology

There are 6000 new cases and 6000 deaths registered in the UK per annum. The peak incidence is 60–80 years with an equal sex distribution. It is a disease of developed countries.

Aetiology

Pancreatic cancer has been associated with:

1. Smoking tobacco.
2. A high coffee consumption.
3. Hereditary pancreatitis.
4. Ataxia telangiectasia.

Pathology

The tumour may be well circumscribed or diffusely infiltrating the pancreas. Thirty per cent arise in the head and are often associated with a dilated common bile duct, and 20 per cent in the body or tail, the remainder being more diffuse in origin.

Carcinoma arises from the ducts (90 per cent) and glandular elements (10 per cent) rather than the hormone-producing cells and is invariably a mucin-producing adenocarcinoma. There may be evidence of a chronic pancreatitis distal to any blocked pancreatic ducts and the majority stain for carcinoembryonic antigen (CEA).

Natural history

The tumour infiltrates diffusely through the gland, or may grow along the pancreatic duct system eventually reaching the common bile duct and ampulla of Vater. The capsule may be breached leading to invasion of the stomach, duodenum, spleen, aorta and retroperitoneal tissues, and transcoelomic spread may occur with diffuse peritoneal involvement and ascites.

Regional lymph nodes are frequently involved and include the pancreaticoduodenal, gastroduodenal, hepatic, superior mesenteric and coeliac groups.

The majority have distant metastases by the time of diagnosis at sites including the liver, lung, skin and brain.

Symptoms

Tumours of the head of the pancreas most frequently present with obstructive jaundice (progressive jaundice, dark urine, pale stools, itching) due to occlusion of the common bile duct. Tumours of the body and tail of the pancreas are more likely to present with pain, usually epigastric with radiation to the back. Extensive pancreatic infiltration or blockage of the major ducts will lead to malabsorption due to exocrine dysfunction, which will result in pale, fatty, offensive stools (steatorrhoea) which float on water and are difficult to flush down the lavatory pan. Pancreatic endocrine dysfunction will lead to impaired glucose tolerance or diabetes mellitus in 20 per cent, causing thirst, polyuria, nocturia and weight loss.

Signs

The patient often has jaundice, and the gallbladder may be palpable in the right upper quadrant of the abdomen suggesting extrahepatic biliary obstruction that is not due to chronic gallstone disease (positive Courvoisier's sign). There will be pale stools on rectal examination and dark urine. Scratch marks on the trunk are a sign of pruritus due to bile salt retention. A mass may be palpable in the epigastrium, fixed due to its retroperitoneal location. Weight loss is common and may lead to profound cachexia. The liver may be enlarged and knobbly consistent with metastatic infiltration. There may be petechiae, purpura and bruising in advanced disease due to disseminated intravascular coagulation (DIC).

Differential diagnosis

Gallstones are a common cause of obstructive jaundice and abdominal pain although they are not commonly associated with systemic symptoms and are not a cause of glucose intolerance.

Investigations

Liver function tests

These will demonstrate the degree of obstructive jaundice, characterized by raised total serum bilirubin, elevated alkaline phosphatase and gammaglutamyltransferase with normal or slightly elevated liver transferases (ALT).

There will be derangement of vitamin K-dependent clotting factors. This will be reflected in a prolongation of the International Normalized Ratio (INR), and will show clinically as bruising and a tendency to prolonged bleeding. A full blood count and clotting profile should always be performed prior to invasive investigations such as an ERCP or CT-guided biopsy, and serum collected for grouping so that fresh frozen plasma or blood can be given at short notice should there be a haemorrhage after biopsy. Patients suspected of having DIC should have blood sent to measure fibrin degradation products (FDPs).

Chest X-ray

A chest X-ray is indicated to exclude pulmonary metastases.

Abdominal ultrasound

This characteristically shows dilatation of the common bile duct associated with a mass lesion in the head of the pancreas, while tumours arising elsewhere in the pancreas will appear as a localized or generalized enlargement of the gland. It is not a sensitive means of demonstrating local invasion or lymphatic involvement, but is useful for excluding liver metastases.

Endoscopic retrograde cholepancreaticogram (ERCP)

A side viewing endoscope is passed into the duodenum allowing cannulation of the ampullary duct under direct vision. Using an image intensifier, a cannula is advanced into the main pancreatic duct and contrast injected to opacify the pancreatic duct system and extrahepatic biliary tree. Gallstones will appear as filling defects in the ducts while pancreatic carcinoma will lead to distortion and obstruction of the pancreatic ducts and extrinsic compression of the common bile duct. Duodenal and pancreatic aspirates collected through the endoscope may be sent for cytology.

Percutaneous transhepatic cholangiography (PTC)

A needle is passed through the skin into a dilated extrahepatic bile duct under ultrasound control and a cholangiogram obtained by injecting contrast into the biliary tree. It will visualize any gallstones in the biliary tree, and in the case of carcinoma confirm blockage of the common bile duct by extrinsic compression at the level of the pancreas.

CT scan of the abdomen

All patients considered suitable for radical surgery should undergo this investigation as it is the best way of defining the extent of local invasion, presence of enlarged regional lymph nodes and liver metastases. It also facilitates a fine needle biopsy when a definitive diagnosis cannot be made by less invasive procedures.

Laparotomy

Occasionally, it is not possible to make a diagnosis from less invasive investigations. If there are no metastases detected during staging and the tumour is otherwise operable, laparotomy is justified with a view to radical surgery if frozen section is positive for malignancy.

Staging

There is no formal staging system in routine clinical use.

Treatment

Radical

Surgery

Patients must be carefully selected for radical surgery as only 10–20 per cent will be suitable candidates. The operation of choice was originally described by Whipple and comprises a pancreaticoduodenectomy although this is associated with a high operative morbidity and mortality, even in the hands of surgeons regularly performing the operation.

Radiotherapy

Carcinoma of the pancreas is incurable using current radiotherapy techniques and doses due to the high incidence of metastases at diagnosis, and the proximity of radiation dose-limiting normal tissues such as the spinal cord, small bowel and kidneys.

Palliative

Surgery

Many patients are found at laparotomy to be inoperable. Rather than going on to perform an operation that stands no chance of prolonging the patient's survival, if the patient has obstructive jaundice or is at risk of developing it in the near future, a bypass procedure (choledochojejunostomy) to allow free drainage of bile is justified. Gastroenterostomy will relieve duodenal obstruction by a large periampullary carcinoma.

Radiotherapy

This is of value in relieving pain due to retroperitoneal tumour extension, but is not a satisfactory treatment for the relief of obstructive jaundice.

Chemotherapy

5-fluorouracil is the most active drug with objective response rates of about 20 per cent, although it is rarely justified to treat patients with pancreatic carcinoma with chemotherapy as most patients will already have systemic symptoms and life expectancy is invariably extremely poor.

Medical treatment

Endoscopic placement of a bile duct stent is of value in relieving obstructive jaundice.

Cholestyramine may relieve the pruritus of intractable obstructive jaundice, while pancreatic enzyme supplements will relieve the steatorrhoea associated with the malabsorption of fats. Vitamin K administered intravenously may be indicated if there is a symptomatic coagulopathy related to a deficiency of the vitamin K-dependent clotting factors.

Tumour-related complications

There are a number of recognized vascular complications:

1. Splenic vein thrombosis – results in portal hypertension and oesophageal varices.
2. Renal vein thrombosis – results in renal congestion and a nephrotic syndrome.
3. Portal vein thrombosis – leads to a Budd–Chiari syndrome characterized by the rapid accumulation of ascites and hepatic congestion.
4. Thrombophlebitis migrans – characterized by intermittent tenderness, erythema and induration of superficial veins.
5. Disseminated intravascular coagulation – mucin production by the tumour leads to activation of the clotting cascade (see Chapter 8).

Non-metastatic manifestations include profound depression, a migratory thrombophlebitis, hypercalcaemia (production of parathyroid hormone-like peptides), Cushing's syndrome (ACTH production), carcinoid syndrome (5HT production), murantic endocarditis and a syndrome of metastatic fat necrosis.

Treatment-related complications

Surgery

Radical pancreaticoduodenectomy has an extremely high operative morbidity and mortality. The loss of exocrine and endocrine pancreatic secretions will lead to permanent diabetes mellitus requiring insulin and malabsorption of fat requiring enzyme supplements with each meal.

Radiotherapy

Radiotherapy to the pancreatic bed will result in temporary anorexia, nausea, vomiting, gastritis, colic and diarrhoea. Late complications are infrequently encountered due to the extremely poor prognosis of the disease.

Prognosis

The outlook is extremely poor with a 5 year survival of less than 5 per cent. Of those undergoing radical surgery, there is a 5 year survival of about 10 per cent.

Rare tumours

Gastrinoma

This is a gastrin-secreting tumour which leads to the Zollinger–Ellison syndrome, characterized by hypersecretion of acid in the stomach leading to intractable peptic ulceration. An elevated serum gastrin level is diagnostic and about half are malignant. It may be associated with adenomata of the pituitary and parathyroid as part of Werner's syndrome (multiple endocrine adenomatosis type 1 – MEA1). After detailed staging with a CT scan and selective venous angiography, the treatment of choice is a partial pancreatectomy.

Carcinoid

This is a rare site for carcinoid, and 5HT production will lead to the carcinoid syndrome (see Chapter 14). Partial pancreatectomy will be curative unless there has been metastasis to the liver.

Insulinoma

This tumour arises from the β cells of the islets and secretes insulin leading to fasting hypoglycaemia. There is an association with MEA1, 90 per cent are benign, 10 per cent multiple, and treatment is surgical as for gastrinoma. Diazoxide is a β cell toxin and relieves the unremitting hypoglycaemia of advanced disease.

Glucagonoma

This arises from the α cells of the pancreas, secretes glucagon, leading to a syndrome of diabetes mellitus, a migratory necrolytic erythema of the skin and stomatitis, and is frequently malignant metastasizing to the liver. Surgery is the treatment of choice but somatostatin and streptozotocin are used for palliation.

Hepatocellular cancer

This is synonymous with hepatoma.

Epidemiology

This is one of the most common tumours worldwide, but is comparatively rare in the UK with 1100 new cases and 700 deaths registered per annum. The peak incidence in the UK is 40–60 years compared with 20–40 years in endemic areas. There is a male to female predominance of 3:2 in the UK. There is a very high incidence in areas where hepatitis B is endemic such as Africa and the Far East.

Aetiology

The hepatitis B virus is implicated, an observation supported by the geographical variation of hepatoma following that of areas where hepatitis B is endemic in the population.

Hepatoma often arises in a cirrhotic liver although the aetiological agent (e.g. alcohol, iron in haemochromatosis, autoantibodies in chronic active hepatitis) responsible for the cirrhosis is unimportant. Macronodular cirrhosis is a greater risk factor than micronodular, and males greatly outnumber females with this complication.

Aflatoxin is a mycotoxin produced by the fungus *Aspergillus flavus* which is found in stored cereals and is a hepatic carcinogen when ingested.

Thorotrast was used as a radiographic contrast agent and contains a high level of the radioactive isotope thorium which emits α particles leading to intense irradiation of the liver which in turn may lead to hepatoma.

Hepatoma has been described in men following use of androgenic anabolic steroids for body building.

Pathology

The tumour grows rapidly, is usually large, arises from the liver parenchyma or a cirrhotic nodule and may be multifocal. In cut section there is bile staining, haemorrhage and necrosis. It invades through the liver capsule, along the hepatic ducts and blood vessels. Intrahepatic ducts proximal to the tumour will be obstructed and therefore dilated.

The tumour is composed of hepatocytes which have lost the characteristic architecture of the portal tracts and frequently stain for α-foetoprotein.

Natural history

The tumour may remain confined to the liver invading along the intrahepatic bile ducts and hepatic veins, or breech the liver capsule leading to invasion of adjacent structures such as the hepatic veins, portal vein, inferior vena cava, right hemidiaphragm, right kidney, right adrenal, stomach and transverse colon.

The hilar lymph nodes at the base of the liver and portal nodes are frequently involved.

The lungs are the most common site of distant metastases although bone, skin and brain may also be involved.

Spread beyond the liver capsule may lead to diffuse peritoneal involvement which in turn may cause malignant ascites.

Symptoms

There is often a long history of increasing ill-health with hepatic pain due to distension of the liver capsule which contains many stretch receptors. The onset of pain may be acute and severe if precipitated by a sudden haemorrhage into the tumour which leads to its rapid enlargement. Swollen legs are a common complaint in advanced cases due to a combination of hypoalbuminaemia and compression of the inferior vena cava. Systemic symptoms such as anorexia, nausea, weight loss, fever and malaise are frequent.

Signs

There may be evidence of an underlying cirrhosis such as clubbing, leuconychia, palmar erythema, jaundice, spider naevi, gynaecomastia, testicular atrophy, ascites, ankle oedema, dilated superficial abdominal wall veins and splenomegaly. Signs of hepatic encephalopathy are rare. The liver may be diffusely enlarged due to cirrhosis, focally enlarged due to the hepatoma or both. An arterial bruit and hepatic rub may be heard over the tumour due to its rich vascular supply and capsular invasion respectively.

Differential diagnosis

A poorly differentiated hepatoma may cause confusion with a carcinoma of unknown primary metastasizing to the liver. A high serum α-foetoprotein (AFP) or positive staining for AFP within a biopsy supports the diagnosis of hepatoma.

Investigations

Liver function tests, clotting profile, serum for grouping:

Liver function derangement is not uncommon but more likely to be due to an underlying cirrhosis rather than the hepatoma itself. Assessment of clotting and blood grouping is necessary prior to liver biopsy or any other invasive procedure.

Serum α-foetoprotein

This is elevated in 90 per cent of cases. It is a useful diagnostic test, of value in monitoring response to therapy (especially surgery) and in predicting relapse.

Chest X-ray

This is mandatory prior to surgery to exclude pulmonary metastases, with a CT scan of the thorax if there is any doubt from the plain radiographs.

Liver ultrasound and percutaneous biopsy

This localizes and measures the tumour, assesses the IVC and other large blood vessels for obstruction, and permits percutaneous biopsy under direct vision. A biopsy of the contralateral lobe is needed in patients for whom resection is planned.

CT scan of the liver and upper abdomen

This complements information obtained from abdominal ultrasound and facilitates percutaneous biopsy when the tumour is not adequately localized by ultrasound. It is mandatory if surgery or radiotherapy is planned.

Laparoscopic biopsy

This is indicated if multiple percutaneous biopsies have failed to give a result.

Angiography

This will define the tumour precisely in terms of its size, position and vascular supply, and is mandatory prior to surgical resection or embolization.

Staging

A formal staging scheme is not in routine clinical use.

Treatment

Radical

Surgery

A major resection of the liver (e.g. lobectomy) is necessary to obtain clearance of tumour, but only 10 per cent of patients will be suitable. Patients requiring more extensive surgery or those with cirrhosis may be considered for hepatectomy and liver transplant. Meticulous pre-operative staging is required whenever such surgery is planned.

Radiotherapy

Several factors make radical radiotherapy impractical:

1. The liver is surrounded by radiosensitive, dose-limiting normal tissues, e.g. stomach, right kidney, small bowel.
2. The liver itself will not tolerate high doses of radiation to a large part of its volume.
3. Hepatoma is a relatively radioresistant tumour.

Palliative

Surgery

Hepatomas derive their blood supply from the hepatic artery and ligation of this vessel close to the liver may palliate local symptoms, particularly pain. The portal vein must be patent to prevent ischaemic necrosis of the liver and a cholecystectomy must be performed lest there be necrosis of the gallbladder. Mortality from this procedure is less than 5 per cent, but the response is short-lived due to development of a collateral tumour circulation.

Radiotherapy

Low doses of radiation may be given with the expectation of relieving hepatic pain.

Chemotherapy

Adriamycin is the most active agent and may be considered in patients symptomatic from metastases.

Hepatic artery embolization

This is less invasive than ligation of the artery, and has a longer symptomatic response as the collateral circulation develops more slowly, and it is anatomically more selective. Unlike ligation, it may be repeated when symptoms recur.

Tumour-related complications

A number of non-metastatic manifestations are recognized including:

1. Hypoglycaemia (insulin-like peptides).
2. Polycythaemia (erythropoietin-like peptides).
3. Hypercalcaemia (parathyroid-like peptides).
4. Feminization (oestrogens).
5. Pyrexia of unknown origin (pyrogens).
6. Porphyria cutanea tarda.

Portal vein thrombosis will lead to splenomegaly, ascites and oesophageal varices, while hepatic vein thrombosis will lead to a Budd–Chiari syndrome with ascites, hepatomegaly and leg oedema. Inferior vena caval obstruction will lead to oedema below the umbilicus. Sudden haemorrhage may occur into the tumour causing acute right upper abdominal pain or into the abdomen causing abdominal pain and distension which may lead to death.

Treatment-related complications

Surgery

Partial hepatectomy may lead to hepatic decompensation if the function of the remaining liver is poor. Transplant patients will also have the problems of rejection and chronic immunosuppression to overcome.

Radiotherapy

Hepatic irradiation invariably causes anorexia, nausea and vomiting during treatment, and radiation hepatitis may result when a large volume of liver has been irradiated.

Hepatic artery embolization

Ectopic embolic phenomena may lead to infarction of other abdominal viscera.

Prognosis

Untreated, most patients die within 1 year. Surgery is the only potentially curative treatment and even after liver transplantation for carefully selected patients, less than 20 per cent will have long-term disease-free survival.

Prevention

Vaccination against hepatitis B, health education and improved food storage should decrease the incidence of hepatoma in endemic areas.

Screening

Measurements of AFP may be performed in cirrhosis patients where the risk of hepatoma is very high (e.g. haemochromatosis) with the hope of detecting hepatoma at a resectable stage.

Rare tumours

Angiosarcoma

This is very rare and associated with medical exposure to thoratrast and industrial exposure to vinyl chloride monomer.

Future prospects

Hepatoma may be amenable to treatment using radioactive isotopes or biological toxins which have been conjugated with antibodies to tumour-specific antigens such as ferritin or AFP. Trials of hepatic artery chemotherapy perfusion are currently in progress.

Cholangiocarcinoma

This is a malignant tumour arising from the epithelium lining the extrahepatic biliary tract.

Epidemiology

This is rare in the UK with less than 1000 new cases and 300 deaths registered per annum. It is about half as common as carcinoma of the gallbladder. The peak incidence is 50–70 years and there is a slight female predominance. It is more common is areas where liver flukes are endemic, e.g. Southeast Asia.

Aetiology

Recognized associations include:

1. Liver flukes, e.g. *Clonorchis sinensis*.
2. Chronic infective cholangitis secondary to gallstones.
3. Ulcerative colitis – a rare complication of chronic inflammatory bowel disease.
4. Radiation – previous use of thoratrast.
5. Congenital biliary abnormalities, e.g. choledochal cyst.

Pathology

Tumours of the upper third of the extrahepatic biliary tree tend to be diffusely sclerosing leading to a malignant stricture. Tumours in the middle third tend to be nodular while those in the lower third tend to be papillary.

   The tumour is usually a well-differentiated mucin-secreting adeno-carcinoma with about half staining for carcinoembryonic antigen (CEA).

Natural history

Tumours of the upper third may infiltrate the liver, while those of the lower third may infiltrate the duodenum and pancreas. Tumours also spread to the hilar, superior mesenteric and coeliac lymph nodes.

   The liver is the most common site of distant metastases although lung and bone may also be involved.

Symptoms

The most common presentation is with obstructive jaundice – jaundice, pruritus, dark urine and pale stools.

Signs

The patient will be jaundiced, the gallbladder may be palpable (positive Courvoisier's sign) and the liver may be congested and therefore smoothly enlarged.

Differential diagnosis

Other causes of obstructive jaundice include:

1. Gallstones.
2. Carcinoma of the head of the pancreas.
3. Benign biliary tract stricture following surgical trauma.
4. Sclerosing cholangitis.

Investigations

Endoscopic retrograde cholepancreaticogram (ERCP – see Carcinoma of the pancreas for a detailed description)

This is the investigation of choice as it will allow an accurate anatomical localization of the tumour, brushings and biliary aspirates for cytology, and therapeutic manoeuvres such as passage of a stent to relieve jaundice.

Percutaneous transhepatic cholangiogram (PTC – see Carcinoma of the pancreas for a detailed description)

This is indicated when ERCP has failed to opacify the biliary tree or adequately display the tumour due to its position.

CT scan of the upper abdomen

This will show the degree of local invasion, any enlarged regional lymph nodes and exclude liver metastases.

Staging

There is no staging system in routine clinical use.

Treatment

Radical

As this is a very rare tumour, the optimum management with radiotherapy and/or surgery is undetermined.

Surgery

This offers the best chance of cure although only 10–20 per cent will be resectable. Tumours of the lower third require pancreaticoduodenectomy, while those with more proximal lesions may be carefully staged and selected for liver transplantation.

Radiotherapy

This tumour is rarely cured by radiotherapy. The difficulties of giving high dose irradiation to this region are lessened by the use of interstitial brachytherapy for localized strictures. A nasobiliary tube is inserted at ERCP or percutaneous tube inserted under ultrasound control, Iridium[192] wire passed down this conduit and left straddling the tumour for 5–7 days. Tumours with extraductal invasion are best treated with external beam irradiation and a brachytherapy boost.

Palliative

Surgery

Choledochojejunostomy will relieve obstructive jaundice in cases not amenable to endoscopic stenting.

Radiotherapy

This is best reserved for palliating pain from local infiltration.

Tumour-related complications

These include:

1. Acute cholangitis – presents with fever, rigors and right upper abdominal pain and usually responds to broad spectrum antibiotics.
2. Secondary biliary cirrhosis – this is caused by chronic cholestasis.

Treatment-related complications

Surgery

The bile duct is a delicate structure prone to stricturing after handling. Biliary fistulae are also a problem after anastomosis.

Radiotherapy

Insertion of a nasobiliary tube and the iridium wire carries a high risk of cholangitis. External beam irradiation carries the same morbidity as outlined for stomach cancer.

Prognosis

The mean survival in untreated cases is only 3 months. Palliative biliary drainage increases this to 9 months while radical radiotherapy gives 2 year survivals of 10–20 per cent.

Carcinoma of the gallbladder

There 1300 new cases and 1000 deaths registered per annum in the UK, with a peak incidence of 60–80 years and a female to male ratio of 3:1. Aetiological factors include:

1. Gallstones – 80 per cent of patients have gallstones, hence the female predominance.
2. Typhoid carriage – there is a greatly increased risk due to carriage of the Salmonella typhi bacteria in the gallbladder which in turn leads to a chronic cholecystitis.

Eighty per cent arise at the fundus or neck of the gallbladder and 90 per cent are adenocarcinomas. The adjacent liver capsule and parenchyma are involved early and there may be lymphatic spread to the hilar nodes around the liver. The liver and lungs are the most common sites for blood-borne metastases.

Many patients are diagnosed incidentally at cholecystectomy and are asymptomatic with no physical signs. Otherwise the presentation resembles benign gallbladder disease with bouts of acute cholecystitis or more chronic and less severe right upper abdominal pain where a mass may be palpable. Staging investigations include liver function tests, chest X-ray, liver ultrasound and a CT scan of the upper abdomen. Treatment comprises cholecystectomy with a wide excision of the surrounding liver and regional lymph node dissection included if there is macroscopic invasion of the liver. Low dose radiotherapy may be of value in relieving pain due to local infiltration, and a biliary drainage procedure will palliate biliary obstruction. The prognosis is poor and the majority of those treated by cholecystectomy alone or a bypass procedure die within 6 months. Of those with liver involvement, 50 per cent die within 3 months of diagnosis and less than 5 per cent survive 1 year.

Carcinoma of the colon and rectum

Epidemiology

There are 27 000 new cases of colorectal cancer and 19 000 deaths registered in the UK per annum and the peak incidence is 60–80 years. For colon cancer, there is a female to male predominance of 4:3, while for rectal cancer there is a male to female predominance of 4:3. It is predominantly a disease of the developed world, being most common in New Zealand, Canada, USA and UK, while rare in Africa, Asia, South America and Japan.

Aetiology

Diet may account for the marked geographical variation in incidence. This is presumed to be due to changes in the bowel flora which produce carcinogens from ingested food, the effect being exacerbated by the slower bowel transit time seen in people taking a low fibre diet. Important dietary factors include:

1. Increased meat consumption.
2. High total fat consumption.
3. High calorie intake.

The incidence has increased in Japan as a Western-style diet has been adopted, and Japanese migrants to the West have subsequently acquired the risk of the indigenous population.

Familial polyposis coli is a dominantly inherited disease characterized by the development of multiple large bowel polyps, one or more of which inevitably undergo malignant change at a young age. Cytogenetic studies in these patients show a loss of tumour suppressor genes on chromosome 5, accounting for the pattern of inheritance observed. Gardener's syndrome is similar to familial polyposis coli but characterized by skeletal and cutaneous abnormalities, e.g. osteomas of the mandible and skull, sebaceous cysts, dermoid cysts. Hereditary non-polyposis cancer accounts for 20 per cent of cases. The relative risk of developing cancer is increased threefold if a first degree relative is afflicted at 45 years and over, and fivefold if 45 years and under. The familial type is also associated with development of carcinoma of the endometrium, ovary, breast and stomach.

Chronic inflammation of the bowel is a rare cause. In the case of ulcerative colitis, the increased risk is related to both the extent and duration of the colitis. Those with disease extending beyond the splenic flexure and/or of more than 10 years' duration being at greatest risk. Chronic Crohn's colitis also confers an increased risk of colorectal cancer.

Pathology

One-third arise in the rectum or rectosigmoid and another third in the sigmoid colon. Most cancers represent malignant change in a benign adenomatous polyp, the highest risk being from villous adenomas, particularly those greater than 2 cm. The tumour may be nodular, ulcerating or diffusely infiltrating, and multiple primaries are found in approximately 5 per cent.

The vast majority are adenocarcinomas (85 per cent glandular, 15 per cent mucinous, 2 per cent signet ring), usually well differentiated, and may show evidence of a preceding benign adenomatous polyp. The tumour cells frequently stain for carcinoembryonic antigen (CEA).

Natural history

The tumour spreads longitudinally and circumferentially along the mucosa, in some cases leading to obstruction of the bowel lumen, and invades deep to the mucosa to infiltrate the muscular wall of the bowel and serosa. Penetration of the serosa leads to direct infiltration of the surrounding abdominal and pelvic viscera, while submucosal spread in the lamina propria may lead to skip lesions well away from the primary tumour. Tumour cells have a propensity to seed in abdominal scars, stomas and even anal fissures, while transcoelomic spread may lead to diffuse peritoneal involvement resulting in ascites and spread to the ovaries.

The regional (mesenteric) lymph nodes may be involved, the likelihood of lymph node metastases increasing with the depth of bowel wall invasion.

The tumour spreads to the liver via the portal circulation, and from there to the lungs, bone, brain and skin.

Symptoms

The tumour most commonly presents with symptoms referable to the large bowel, 20 per cent presenting as a surgical emergency with acute bowel obstruction or peritonitis due to perforation. In the remainder there is usually a history of one or more of the following:

1. Change in bowel habit – may be an increase or decrease in frequency of defaecation or a change in stool consistency, alternating diarrhoea and constipation being highly suspicious of cancer.
2. Blood per rectum – varies in quantity depending on degree of tumour ulceration and/or vascularity. The blood will be bright red and more likely streaked on the outside of the stool if the tumour arises in rectum or sigmoid, or dark red and mixed in with the stool if the tumour arises more proximally in the colon.
3. Mucus per rectum – more likely to be noticed with distal lesions, particularly those of a mucinous variety.
4. Tenesmus – the patient has a frequent urge to defaecate but passes little stool on each occasion. This is usually seen in rectal tumours, particularly if bulky or invading deeply.
5. Obstructive symptoms – characterized by intermittent colicky abdominal pain. It is more common in tumours of the descending colon where the faeces are more solid compared with left colon tumours where the stool is more liquid.
6. Anaemia – chronic bleeding leads to iron deficiency. It is a particular feature of right-sided colonic tumours which have few associated gastrointestinal symptoms.

Signs

The primary tumour may be palpable by digital examination of the rectum as a circumscribed area of mucosal induration, often with irregular heaped-up margins and a friable ulcer base which bleeds on contact. Proximal tumours may be palpable in the pouch of Douglas per vaginam, and caecal tumours may be palpable by abdominal examination. Signs indicative of spread outside the pelvis include:

1. Troisier's sign due to enlargement of Virchow's lymph node in the left supraclavicular fossa.
2. Ascites indicating peritoneal involvement.
3. Hepatomegaly suggesting possible liver metastases.

Rarely, locally advanced disease in the pelvis may lead to formation of a fistula between the adjacent bladder (colovesical – suggested by faecal debris in the urine or pneumaturia) or vagina (colovaginal – suggested by leakage of faeces per vaginam).

Investigations

Digital examination of the rectum/vagina

This permits evaluation of the site, size and extent of local invasion of tumours of the rectum.

Proctoscopy and sigmoidoscopy

This is mandatory to exclude a second primary tumour of the distal 25 cm of the large bowel, and in the case of a rectal primary allows accurate assessment of distance of lesion from anal verge and permits biopsy to obtain a tissue diagnosis.

Double contrast barium enema

This is a very sensitive and specific investigation which can detect tumours 1 cm or more and should be performed in all cases. It allows rapid assessment of the large bowel from the rectum to the caecum and can detect synchronous primaries or benign polyps elsewhere. Carcinomas appear as irregular mass lesions with an ulcerating centre, and if circumferential give rise to a characteristic 'apple core' stricture.

Flexible sigmoidoscopy

This visualizes tumours of the distal 50–60 cm of the large bowel and is better tolerated than colonoscopy for biopsy of such lesions.

Colonoscopy

This facilitates a detailed survey of the whole large bowel, is more sensitive than a barium enema and is useful for biopsying tumours of the transverse and ascending colon.

Other mandatory investigations include:

1. Full blood count to exclude anaemia.
2. Liver function tests and liver ultrasound as a screen for liver metastases.
3. Chest X-ray to exclude lung metastases.

Staging

Clinicopathological staging according to Duke:

A – Confined to the bowel wall.
B – Tumour has breached the bowel wall.
C – Regional lymph node involvement.
D – Distant metastases.

Management

Radical

Surgery

This is the only curative treatment modality. Eighty per cent of all tumours are resectable. Prior to resection of the primary tumour, a detailed inspection and palpation of the open abdomen and pelvis is performed to document the exact extent of disease, with special reference to the liver, and suspicious tissues should be biopsied if not part of the main resection. Tumours of the colon are treated by hemicolectomy, while those of the rectum are treated by an anterior resection. Abdominoperineal resection may be required for the lowest rectal tumours, but in many cases can be avoided with current surgical techniques. In each case, the mesentery containing the regional lymph nodes is also resected.

Radiotherapy

Moderate doses of radiation prior to surgery may be of use in converting an inoperable tumour to one that is operable, and thereby offer a chance of a curative approach to treatment. There is also evidence to suggest that pre-operative radiotherapy is of value in patients with operable Duke's C disease.

Similarly, there is evidence that post-operative radiotherapy to the region of the primary tumour decreases the risk of local recurrence in patients with Duke's C carcinoma of the rectum by about 25 per cent but no effect on colonic cancers is seen and there is no benefit in terms of prolongation of survival.

Radiation given with curative intent in inoperable cases is limited by the close proximity to radiosensitive normal tissues which makes it very difficult to give a tumouricidal dose. There is also a high incidence of occult metastases in this group which limits the treatment outcome.

Chemotherapy

The most active chemotherapy agent in colorectal cancer is 5-fluorouracil (5FU) with response rates of 15–25 per cent in metastatic disease. There is little benefit in adding other chemotherapy agents, although in recent years it has become apparent that improved response rates can be seen when 5FU is 'modulated' by combining it with calcium leucovorin (folinic acid) which enhances the inhibition of the enzyme thymidylate synthetase required by the cancer cells to produce DNA and proliferate.

Despite an 80 per cent resection rate, almost half of such patients will have a relapse of their disease in the liver, usually within 2 years of surgery. Much effort has therefore been put into assessing the role of adjuvant chemotherapy to eradicate the micrometastases which have been shed from the tumour prior to or during its resection. Patients who have had surgery for Duke's B and C tumours and have clear surgical margins may benefit from 1 year's adjuvant therapy with 5FU and the immunostimulatory agent levamisole, with significant prolongation of disease-free survival and overall survival. However, such treatment is not widely accepted in the UK at present. The results of similar studies using 5FU and leucovorin are awaited. The role of perioperative portal vein infusions of 5FU is also under investigation following reports of prolonged disease-free and overall survivals with this approach.

Palliative

Surgery

If the tumour is inoperable, a bypass procedure or defunctioning colostomy may be of value in alleviating symptoms. Of those with liver metastases only 5 per cent are amenable to resection of the metastases, with 20–30 per cent 5 year survival in those with solitary metastases or multiple metastases limited to a single lobe of the liver.

Radiotherapy

This is of benefit in inoperable disease, local recurrence after surgery and symptomatic metastases. It is very effective in relieving bleeding, mucorrhoea and local pain, with response rates of about 75 per cent. Symptomatic presacral recurrence is a particular problem after surgery (Fig. 9.2) and can be helped greatly by radiotherapy.

Chemotherapy

For the palliation of metastatic disease, continuously infused 5FU produces superior response rates to bolus doses. Addition of leucovorin improves the response rate to 30–40 per cent, but the median duration of response is about 10 months.

Fig. 9.2   Pelvic CT scan showing presacral recurrence of a colonic cancer.

Prognosis

Duke staging and operability are the most important prognostic factors. The 5 year survivals are 80 per cent, 60 per cent and 30 per cent for Duke's A, B and C tumours respectively.

Screening

Even for symptomatic individuals, screening is expensive and un-rewarding as gastrointestinal symptoms have a low positive predictive value for cancer. However, regular faecal occult blood testing followed by colonoscopy for positive tests does significantly increase the proportion of Duke's A cancers detected. The cost of such screening has been estimated at £2000 per detected cancer. High risk groups require regular colonoscopy, in particular those with familial polyposis coli and long-standing, extensive ulcerative colitis.

Carcinoma of the anus

Epidemiology

This is a rare tumour with only 300 new cases and 200 deaths registered in England and Wales per annum. It comprises about 4 per cent of large bowel tumours with a peak incidence of 50–70 years and a slight female predominance overall. Anal margin tumours are more common in men; anal canal tumours are more common in women.

Aetiology

Homosexual activity, in particular ano-receptive intercourse, is associated with anal cancer, and there is evidence that this is due to transmission of the human papilloma virus types 16 and 18, 50 per cent of cancer sufferers testing positive for these which is analogous with carcinoma of the cervix. There is also evidence among attenders to sexually transmitted disease (STD) clinics that up to 60 per cent of homosexuals will have asymptomatic anal intraepithelial neoplasia (AIN) which is comparable to cervical intraepithelial neoplasia (CIN).

Pathology

The tumour may arise from skin at the anal margin or from the anal canal, appearing as a nodule, polyp or ulcer with everted edges.

Ninety per cent are squamous carcinomas, most of the remainder adenocarcinomas arising from mucous glands. Anal margin tumours are well differentiated as they are akin to squamous carcinomas of the skin, whereas 75 per cent of anal canal tumours are poorly differentiated. There may be *in situ* carcinoma in the surrounding epithelium.

Natural history

The tumour will spread circumferentially and longitudinally within the anus and may invade the lower rectum or perianal skin. Deeper infiltration leads to involvement of the sphincters, ischiorectal fossae, vagina and urethra.

Lymphatic spread occurs in 10 per cent and is more common with anal canal tumours. The first station lymph nodes are the inguinal groups from which there may be spread to the iliac nodes. Involvement of the distal rectum may lead to infiltration of the inferior mesenteric nodes.

Haematogenous spread is very uncommon at presentation. Sites of distant metastases include the liver, lungs and skeleton.

Symptoms

Patients present with anal symptoms such as discharge, irritation, bleeding or tenesmus.

Signs

Tumours of the anal verge or most distal part of the anal canal should be easily seen on parting the buttocks. The tumour should be papable as an indurated ulcer or nodule on digital examination. Enlarged inguinal nodes should be sought although a proportion of enlarged nodes will be secondary to infection.

Differential diagnosis

This includes:

1. Sexually transmitted diseases – syphilis may present in a homosexual male as a painless perianal ulcer. This can be confirmed by serology and the presence of Treponemes.

2. Genital warts – these may be confused with a papilliform, well-differentiated carcinoma.
3. Crohn's disease of the anus.
4. Basal cell carcinoma.

Investigations

Proctoscopy

This is an essential investigation, permitting the tumour to be visualized directly and biopsied, and complements the findings of a digital rectal examination.

Examination under anaesthetic (EUA)

This is the best staging investigation in an anxious or uncooperative patient. In a woman, a full bimanual examination is mandatory to assess the extent of local spread. An EUA will also permit the taking of a generous biopsy with minimal distress and discomfort.

CT scan of the pelvis

This permits an assessment of the degree of deep invasion of the tumour and is of value in excluding pelvic lymphadenopathy when the inguinal nodes are involved.

Fine needle aspiration of any enlarged inguinal lymph nodes

This will confirm the presence of any carcinoma cells within the nodes which is important in planning management.

Other mandatory investigations

These include:

1. Liver function tests and liver ultrasound as a screen for liver metastases.
2. Chest X-ray to exclude lung metastases.

Staging

T1 – tumour 2 cm or less in greatest dimension.
T2 – tumour > 2 cm but not > 5cm in greatest dimension.
T3 – tumour > 5 cm in greatest dimension.
T4 – tumour of any size with extension to other neighbouring structures, e.g. vagina, urethra, bladder.

Treatment

Radical

Surgery

Anal margin tumours may be treated by wide local excision alone, with more extensive surgery reserved for salvage of local relapse. In anal canal tumours, an abdominoperineal resection (APR) is necessary which will result in the patient having a permanent colostomy. Pre-operative conselling by a stomatherapist should be arranged in all patients in whom an APR is planned. Patients with cytologically positive inguinal nodes should undergo a block dissection of the groins.

Radiotherapy

This has the advantage of allowing sphincter preservation, and local recurrences can still be salvaged by an APR. Radiotherapy is initially given to the pelvis and inguinal nodes bilaterally over 4 weeks followed by a boost dose of radiation to the anal tumour alone, either by external beam radiation or by interstitial brachytherapy (Fig. 9.3), with a further boost to the inguinal region if there are involved nodes. A poor objective response after the initial phase of radiotherapy is an indication to proceed to APR.

Fig. 9.3 Implant of small bore tubes around the anus which will be loaded with radioactive iridium wire.

Chemotherapy

5-fluorouracil and mitomycin C are currently being used in combination with high dose radiotherapy in an attempt to increase the complete response rate. Increased gastrointestinal morbidity can be expected with combined modality treatment, particularly diarrhoea.

Palliative

Surgery

In the exceptional case of a very advanced inoperable tumour leading to anal occlusion, a defunctioning colostomy may be justified.

Radiotherapy

Pelvic/perineal radiotherapy may be used to palliate symptomatic local recurrence after radical surgery.

Tumour-related complications

An advanced tumour may lead to an aberrant connection between the anal canal and the perineum, vagina or urethra leading to faecal incontinence. The ischiorectal fossae are anatomically close to the anus and particularly prone to secondary infection and abscess formation.

Treatment-related complications

Radiotherapy

The perianal region does not tolerate radiotherapy well as the skin is constantly subjected to friction when sitting and walking, trauma when patients are having to defaecate frequently, moisture due to sweating and perhaps discharge from the anus. During radiotherapy the patient can be expected to experience diarrhoea, tenesmus and perianal irritation/soreness. These symptoms will begin 1–2 weeks after starting radiotherapy and persist for 1–4 weeks after it has finished. In the longer term, chronic proctocolitis may manifest as diarrhoea, tenesmus, bleeding and mucus per rectum which can be treated conservatively with topical steroids. High doses of radiation to the groins may lead to occlusion of the lymphatics leading to chronic lymphoedema which is best managed with pressure garments.

Surgery

The main morbidity in the short term is from dehiscence of the perineal wound and pelvic infection. Extensive pelvic surgery such as an abdominoperineal resection may damage autonomic nerves leading to urinary incontinence and impotence in men. The psychosexual trauma and effect on body image may be considerable.

Chemotherapy

Apart from the usual complications from these chemotherapy drugs, the combination of radiotherapy and chemotherapy leads to severe gastrointestinal toxicity causing anorexia, nausea, vomiting and diarrhoea.

Prognosis

The overall 5 year survival is 70 per cent, patients with anal margin tumours faring better than those with anal canal tumours.

Screening/prevention

The high incidence of AIN in STD clinics may make screening a worthwhile exercise in this small group, particularly in homosexuals.

Rare tumours

Melanoma

These present late and have a much poorer prognosis than cutaneous melanomas.

10

Urological cancer

Kidney

Renal cell carcinoma (hypernephroma)

Epidemiology

This accounts for 2 per cent of all malignancies with around 3600 cases each year in the UK. It is slightly more common in males than females. The incidence is high in Europe, particularly Denmark, and lowest in Japan.

Aetiology

Smoking. Cadmium exposure may also be a factor.

Pathology

Tumours may arise from any part of the renal tissue – one-quarter involve the whole kidney, one-third the upper pole, and one-third the lower pole.

Macroscopically the tumour is usually solid, expanding the renal tissue with a central area of necrosis or cystic degeneration and other haemorrhagic areas. Occasionally a tumour may arise within the wall of a cyst.

Renal cell tumours are thought to arise from the lining cells of the proximal convoluted tubule. Microscopically they are adenocarcinomas composed of characteristic clear cells although the degree of differentiation can vary from a well-differentiated tumour to a highly anaplastic appearance.

Natural history

The tumour invades the surrounding kidney and may grow into the renal vein and thence into the inferior vena cava (IVC).

Lymph node spread involves the renal hilar nodes and progresses to the para-aortic chain.

Blood-borne metastases characteristically go to the lung and bone although many other sites including skin, central nervous system and liver are also recognized.

Spontaneous regression of metastases, typically lung deposits monitored on chest X-ray, is often referred to in the context of renal cell cancer.

While such events undoubtedly occur the true incidence is extremely low, the verified incidence being around 7 per cent of patients with metastatic disease. Spontaneous regression of the primary tumour is virtually unknown.

Symptoms

Haematuria, typically painless, is the most common presenting symptom.

Loin pain may occur acutely due to haemorrhage within the tumour or chronically as the tumour enlarges.

Symptoms of metastases may be present, in particular bone pain or even pathological fracture (bone metastases) and cough with or without haemoptysis (lung metastases).

Symptoms of paraneoplastic conditions, associated with renal cell cancer, may be present, which include hypercalcaemia and polycythaemia.

There may also be general symptoms of malignancy such as malaise anorexia and weight loss.

Signs

The primary tumour may be palpable as a mass in the loin, and in 10–20 per cent of patients there is associated fever.

Differential diagnosis

Other causes of haematuria should be considered, in particular benign renal adenomas, tumours of the renal pelvis, renal tract stones and bladder tumours.

Other causes of loin pain which should be taken into account, include renal stones or hydronephrosis.

Investigations

A full blood count may show anaemia due to chronic haematuria or polycythaemia due to tumour production of erythyropoeitin-like substances. Serum calcium may be raised, and a chest X-ray may show typical 'cannon-ball' metastases.

The renal tumour will be imaged on both ultrasound or CT scan. The latter will also give information on renal vein/IVC invasion and involvement of surrounding structures. The role of IVU where CT is widely available is debatable. Figure 10.1 shows the appearance of a renal carcinoma on CT scan.

Tissue diagnosis may be obtained by fine needle aspirate cytology or biopsy.

Isotope bone scans are not routinely recommended but X-ray skeletal survey may be of value. The typical lytic bone lesions of renal cell carcinoma may give false negative bone scan images.

Fig. 10.1 CT scan demonstrating a large renal carcinoma arising from the right kidney.

Staging

Full TNM staging is not often used in the clinical assessment of renal cell cancers. Important features are the size of the primary tumour and involvement of surrounding structures including the renal vein which will determine operability of the primary, and the presence of distant metastases.

Treatment

Surgery

Radical nephrectomy in which the perirenal fat, perirenal fascia, adrenal gland and regional nodes are removed en bloc is the operation of choice with superior local control rates to simple nephrectomy. Tumour invading the renal vein can be successfully removed and this is therefore not an absolute contraindication to radical treatment.

Transarterial embolization pre-operatively has been used in the past to improve the operability of large tumours. There is no good evidence that this is translated into better survival.

Radiotherapy

Pre- or post-operative radiotherapy is sometimes given electively or in the post-operative setting where there has been incomplete surgical clearance.

Palliative treatment

Local irradiation of bone metastases is required.

Brain metastases may benefit from cranial irradiation.

Lung metastases do not usually lend themselves to local irradiation, however, in the occasional patient who presents some years after treatment of the primary tumour with a solitary lung metastasis; surgical excision may be appropriate, accompanied by a further long disease-free period if not cure. A similar approach to solitary brain metastases may also be applied.

There is no effective chemotherapy for renal cell cancer.

Hormone responses occur with progestogens although the true response rate is probably quite low, perhaps less than 10 per cent.

Biological agents such as interferon and interleukin 2 (IL2) are active against renal cancer; response rates of around 15 per cent are seen with interferon and 20–30 per cent with IL2 particularly if administered with lymphokine-activated killer T lymphocytes (LAK cells). However, the true benefit for the patient with metastatic renal cell carcinoma from such treatments, which are themselves associated with side effects, remains uncertain.

Tumour-related complications

- Hypercalcaemia.
- Polycythaemia.

Renal function is usually unaffected provided the contralateral kidney is normal.

Prognosis

The prognosis for tumour localized to the kidney is good with 5 year survival after radical nephrectomy of around 50 per cent.

Even in the presence of metastases renal cell cancer often has a long and indolent course so that 5–10 per cent of patients with lung metastases will survive for 5 years or more.

Screening and future prospects

Simple urinalysis for microscopic haematuria and cytology are readily available. However, while sensitive it is non-specific and results in unacceptably high false positive rates for routine application.

It is of interest that this tumour is one of the few to show responses to the biological response-modifying agents and future developments in this area may well lead to further new treatments.

Prostate

Epidemiology

The incidence of prostate cancer is rising. This may reflect an increasing proportion of the population over 70 years, a greater diagnostic rate and possibly a true increase in incidence in younger men.

There are around 10 800 cases in the UK each year with an incidence of 19 in 100 000 compared to 91 in 100 000 in US black men, 51 in 100 000 in

US white men and 6 in 100 000 in Japan. In the UK it ranks third behind lung and large bowel cancer for deaths from cancer.

Aetiology

Age

Rare under 45 years but increases with age being almost universal at post-mortem in men aged over 80 years.

Sexual activity

More common in married men, related to the number of sexual partners, frequency of sexual activity and a history of sexually transmitted disease. A positive correlation with circulating testosterone levels and a negative correlation with oestrogen levels has been claimed.

Familial

Particularly in young men under 45 years with first degree relatives affected. Benign prostatic hypertrophy is often also present, but no direct causal relationship has been demonstrated.

It is more common in city dwellers than rural communities, and is associated with a high fat and meat diet, and an occupational exposure to cadmium.

Pathology

Cancer of the prostate develops most commonly in the peripheral part of the gland, this accounting for 70 per cent while only 10 per cent arise centrally. The remainder arise in the transitional zone. Eighty-five per cent are diffuse multifocal tumours.

Microscopically prostate cancer is typically an adenocarcinoma of varying differentiation. Various grading systems based on morphological appearances have been described, all of which correlate with outcome low grade tumours (grade 0 or 1) having a good prognosis and high grade tumours (usually designated grade 3 or 4) having a poor prognosis. The commonly used system is that of Gaeta using grades 1 to 4 which is an adaptation of the Gleason score.

Where there is doubt as to the primary origin of a tumour deposit, a prostatic primary will be characterized by staining for acid phosphatase. Androgen and progestogen receptors have been demonstrated on the surface of prostate cancer cells although the value of this in routine clinical use remains uncertain.

Natural history

Local growth results in infiltration of the prostate gland and surrounding tissues, particularly into the seminal vesicles.

Lymph node metastases are not often prominent in the clinical course of the disease but are not infrequent if looked for by lymphangiogram or by CT scan, being demonstrated in 20–30 per cent of patients with disease clinically localized to the prostate gland.

Distant spread is predominantly blood borne typically by retrograde venous spread through the vertebral plexus of veins so that bone metastases to the spine are common although all parts of the skeleton may be affected. This is demonstrated in Figure 10.2.

Soft tissue metastases, e.g. lung or liver, although well recognized are uncommon in prostatic cancer.

Symptoms

Prostate cancer is often asymptomatic and found either at post-mortem or incidentally during the investigation of another condition.

Prostatic outflow obstructive symptoms are common with frequency, poor stream, nocturia and terminal dribble.

Many cases of prostate cancer present with symptoms of bone metastases with either bone pain or less often spinal cord compression.

Hypercalcaemia may occur.

General symptoms of malignancy including malaise, anorexia and weight loss may also be present.

Signs

Tumours are usually palpable per rectum as a hard nodule or diffusely infiltrating abnormality which in more advanced cases may be palpable invading surrounding pelvic tissues. Typically there is loss of the midline sulcus of the gland which is present in the normal or hypertrophied prostate.

Bone metastases may be clinically apparent when complicated by pain, pathological fracture or neurological signs.

Differential diagnosis

Benign prostatic hypertrophy.

Investigations

A full blood count may show a reduction of haemoglobin, white cells or platelets with widespread bone metastases.

Hypercalcaemia and uraemia should be excluded on routine biochemistry.

IVU will demonstrate the enlarged gland indenting the bladder and any associated hydronephrosis.

CT scan gives more detail of surrounding soft tissue, in particular seminal vesical invasion and lymph node enlargement.

Transrectal ultrasound is the most sensitive means of assessing the prostate gland and may be used to direct needle biopsy towards suspicious areas of the gland.

Serum acid phosphatase will be raised in metastatic disease.

Prostate-specific antigen is measured in the blood and is more specific than acid phosphatase for diagnosis and monitoring of the disease although it may be slightly elevated (up to 10 ng/ml) in benign prostatic hypertrophy.

Isotope bone scan is essential to exclude bone metastases. A positive scan is shown in Figure 10.2.

Diagnosis is made either at transurethral resection of the prostate (TURP) or on needle biopsy per rectum. There is evidence that TURP is associated with a higher incidence of subsequent dissemination and therefore simple needle biopsy is to be preferred in the absence of other indications for TUR.

Fig 10.2 Isotope bone scan demonstrating multiple areas of increased isotope uptake due to bone metastases from carcinoma of the prostate.

Staging

Staging of cancer of the prostate is a little confused because of the existence of two different systems, the TNM system and the Jewitt system widely adopted in the US. The two systems are shown in Table 10.1. The important principles are to distinguish early localized carcinoma of the prostate from locally extensive disease from that which has already metastasized.

Treatment

Radical treatment is indicated for prostatic cancer which is localized to the prostate gland or immediate structures with no evidence on the basis

Table 10.1   Staging of prostatic cancer

TNM	Jewitt	
T0	A1, A2	Asymptomatic
T1		incidental finding
T2	B1, B2	Confined within capsule of gland
T3	C1, C2	Extension beyond capsule of gland
T4		
N1, N2, N3	D1	Involvement of regional nodes
M1	D2	Distant metastases

of isotope bone scan or serum acid phosphatase/prostate-specific antigen of distant metastases.

Radical prostatectomy

This is indicated for disease that is localized to the gland, i.e. stages T1 and T2.

The operation involves removal of the entire prostate and adjacent bladder neck, both seminal vesicles, the vasa deferentia and surrounding fascia. It requires considerable expertise and only a small number of urological surgeons in the UK perform this procedure although it is widespread in the US. Complications include erectile impotence and occasional urinary incontinence.

Radical radiotherapy

This is indicated for all patients with disease localized to the pelvis. There is no evidence that prophylactic treatment of pelvic lymph nodes is of value and a small treatment volume encompassing known disease in the prostate and seminal vesicles is adequate. Localization with CT scanning greatly increases the accuracy of treatment. Side effects include bowel and bladder irritation but in the majority of patients potency is preserved.

Hormone therapy by androgen deprivation or blockade is effective in most patients, usually reserved for relapse or those presenting with metastatic disease.

Palliative treatment

For metastatic disease hormone therapy will achieve a response in 70–80 per cent.

Hormone therapy may be given in a number of forms shown in Table 10.2, all of which are equally effective and the choice will in general be based on patient acceptability and availability.

First line treatment for a patient presenting with metastatic prostate cancer will generally be either cyproterone acetate or an injection of a gonadotrophin-releasing hormone (GnRH) agonist. Around 80 per cent of

Table 10.2 Hormone therapy for prostate cancer

Bilateral orchidectomy	Anti-androgen drugs	GnRH analogue
Surgical procedure	Oral medication	Monthly injection
Permanent	Reversible	Reversible
Compliance guaranteed	Tablets may be missed	Compliance guaranteed if injection given
Patient acceptance variable	Readily accepted	Readily accepted

Anti-androgen drugs include cyproterone acetate and flutamide. Stilboestrol has been used in the past but is limited by excessive cardiovascular side effects. Gonadotrophin releasing hormone (GnRH) analogue drugs include goserelin and leuprorelin.

patients will respond to this manoeuvre. Permanent androgen deprivation by orchidectomy may then be offered to responders with the alternative of continuing with medical treatment.

Patients will inevitably relapse despite an initial response, the median duration of response being around 18 months. Unfortunately response to a second hormone manoeuvre is usually disappointing and further treatment will be based on control of specific symptoms.

There is no effective chemotherapy for prostatic cancer and outside clinical trials this will not form part of the patient's management.

Other palliative treatments which will be of value in these patients include the appropriate use of analgesics and coanalgesics for bone pain, palliative radiotherapy for bone pain or neurological complications and the management of hypercalcaemia.

Tumour-related complications

- Obstructive hydronephrosis.
- Hypercalcaemia.
- Spinal cord compression.

Treatment-related complications

Surgery

Impotence and urinary incontinence.

Radiotherapy

Bowel and bladder damage.

Hormone therapy

Impotence.

Prognosis

While agressive forms of prostatic cancer are recognized, particularly in young men, in the majority of cases the natural history of the disease will span several years. Because of this it is difficult to judge the results of treatment on short-term survival figures.

Untreated, localized carcinoma of the prostate will still give a 5 year survival of 80 per cent although many will have locally progressive disease. After radical treatment, surgical or radiotherapeutic, 10 year survivals in excess of 80 per cent are to be expected, falling to around 50 per cent for disease extending outside the capsule of the gland.

Patients presenting with metastastic disease have a median survival of 18 to 24 months.

Screening

Digital rectal examination, serum PSA and transrectal ultrasound offer a high chance of detecting pre-clinical prostate cancer. Extensive studies are currently underway in Europe to evaluate the effect of screening healthy men and this is already common practice in the US, where 50 per cent of prostate cancers are detected while still localized to the gland compared to only 10 per cent in the UK.

Rarer tumours

Transitional cell tumours of the prostate arising from the urethra usually present and are managed in the same way as other urothelial tumours.

Bladder

Epidemiology

There are around 10 000 cases of bladder cancer in the UK each year. It is twice as common in men as in women and is unusual under the age of 50 years, being most common in the 70s and 80s.

Aetiology

Chemical carcinogens

These include aniline dyes; rubber industry by-products such as beta-naphthylamine and benzidine; and drugs – exposure to excessive amounts of phenacetin or cyclophosphamide.

Smoking

Chronic irritation

This is related to bladder diverticulae and infection with schistosomiasis is also important, the latter being associated with squamous carcinomas in younger age groups.

Pathology

Macroscopically bladder cancer can appear as papillary or solid lesions and may be solitary or more usually multiple. The usual area of the bladder affected is the lateral wall and involvement of the bladder base is also common.

Microscopically the majority of cancers are transitional cell tumours of varying differentiation graded from well to poorly differentiated using a numerical scale G1 to G3. These account for 90 per cent of all bladder cancers. Of the remainder 7 per cent are squamous carcinomas and 3 per cent are adenocarcinomas.

Natural history

Most bladder cancers probably arise as fairly indolent papillomas which left untreated progress both in terms of dedifferentiation and local invasion. The primary tumour invades locally into the bladder muscle wall and thence into perivesical fat.

Lymphatic spread involves pelvic lymph nodes and then para-aortic nodes.

Blood-borne metastases particularly arise in lungs and bone.

In many if not all patients there is a generalized instability of the urothelium and a risk of further tumours developing not only elsewhere in the bladder but also throughout the ureters and renal pelvises. Biopsies of adjacent sites frequently demonstrate dysplasia and a clinical picture of multiple recurrent transitional cell tumours throughout the tract is well recognized.

Symptoms

Painless haematuria and other urinary symptoms such as frequency, urgency and dysuria may be present.

Metastases may cause cough, haemoptysis or bone pain but this is an unusual presentation of bladder cancer.

General symptoms of malaise, anorexia and weight loss may also be present.

Signs

In most patients there will be no clinical signs of bladder cancer. Bladder tumours are rarely palpable per rectum or per vaginam and only in advanced cases will a suprapubic mass be palpable.

Differential diagnosis

Other causes of haematuria should be considered including urinary tract infection, stones and renal tumours.

Investigations

Routine blood investigations may reveal anaemia due to chronic haematuria and renal impairment if there is obstructive hydronephrosis.

Chest X-ray will demonstrate metastases if present.

Urine cytology may reveal malignant cells and is a useful screening test. Negative urinalysis, however, should not exclude further investigations.

IVU may demonstrate a filling defect in the bladder and renal tract obstruction if present. It is also important to exclude tumours in other parts of the urinary tract since a generalized instability of the urothelium is often present with multiple tumours developing between the renal pelvis and the urethra.

Cystoscopy is the definitive investigation at which mucosal abnormalities can be carefully documented and biopsies taken. Transurethral resection of bladder tumour (TURB) can also be performed during the course of this.

CT scan will demonstrate extravesical extension of tumour and lymph node enlargement if present.

Staging

The TNM staging system is commonly used, as shown in Table 10.3. The important features in deciding on appropriate therapy are the extent of local invasion into the bladder wall, tumour differentiation and distant spread.

Treatment

Local resection

Transurethral resection is performed for superficial (T1) bladder tumours followed by careful cystoscopic surveillance.

Table 10.3   TNM staging of bladder cancer

Tis	*In situ* carcinoma
T1	Superficial invasive carcinoma confined to subepithelial connective tissue
T2	Invasion of superficial muscle
T3	Invasion of deep muscle
T3a	Within bladder wall
T3b	Extension to perivesical fat
T4a	Invasion of surrounding pelvic structures
T4b	Distant metastases

Recurrence will occur in around 50 per cent and progression to a higher stage or worse grade will occur in around 15 per cent. This is particularly the case in large tumours, high grade tumours and those with multiple areas of mucosal dysplasia or frank malignancy. In patients who fail initial resection further local resection may be attempted. Where there are multiple recurrences and when there is progression to a high grade tumour then alternative therapies may be required.

Intravesical chemotherapy

This will improve local control of superficial bladder cancer. Various agents have been used including adriamycin, thiotepa and mitomycin C. More recently BCG has been used and may give better results although a higher incidence of local complications and pulmonary infection is also reported. The use of other immunotherapeutic agents including interferon, tumour necrosis factor and IL2 is also under investigation.

Radical radiotherapy

This may take the form of an interstitial implant for localized superficial bladder tumours or more usually radical external beam treatment. This is indicated for progressive high grade T1 tumours and as initial treatment for T2 and T3 tumours.

Pre-operative radiotherapy may be selected for patients undergoing primary surgery for invasive bladder cancer.

Cystectomy

This may be considered for progressive superficial bladder cancer and recurrence after radical radiotherapy. There is some evidence that elective pre-operative radiotherapy improves results compared to surgery alone as primary treatment for invasive bladder cancer. It is also used to salvage radical cystectomy and involves removal of the bladder and perivesical tissues together with pelvic lymphadenectomy. For multifocal lesions urethrectomy is also recommended. Urine is diverted via an ileal conduit to the abdominal wall.

Partial cystectomy is occasionally used for a localized superficial tumour or where there is only minimal muscle invasion.

There are two prevailing philosophies in the treatment of invasive bladder cancer. Many centres offer all patients radical radiotherapy and reserve surgery for salvage. This approach results in initial bladder preservation and complete regression of the bladder tumour in around 60 per cent but local recurrence requiring salvage surgery may occur in over half of these. The alternative approach is to offer selected patients, particularly those under 65 years, pre-operative radiotherapy and elective cystectomy with which 5 year survivals of around 35 per cent are to be expected, although without bladder preservation. No survival advantage between these two approaches has become apparent.

Chemotherapy

Bladder cancer is sensitive to chemotherapy. Currently drug combinations such as CMV (cisplatinum, methotrexate and vinblastine) are used with which response rates of 50–60 per cent may be achieved, some of which are complete responses. The role of chemotherapy in the routine management of bladder cancer has yet to be fully defined and studies are seeking to evaluate such schedules as adjuvant treatment in combination with radical local treatment.

Palliative treatment

This may be required for locally advanced tumours or in the frail and elderly who cannot tolerate radical treatment. Local radiotherapy will help haematuria and local pain, given in short low dose schedules over 1 or 2 weeks.

Tumour-related complications

* Haematuria leading to clot retention and clot colic.
* Ureteric obstruction leading to hydronephrosis and renal failure.

Treatment-related complications

Surgery

Cystectomy has an operative mortality particularly in the elderly. Stoma problems may arise and impotence occurs.

Radiotherapy

This may result in both bowel and bladder damage.

Prognosis

Ten year cause-specific survival ranges from around 70 per cent for T1 bladder cancer to 20 per cent for T3 and less than 5 per cent for T4 tumours.

Screening

Urine cytology is currently in use for patients at high risk by virtue of industrial exposure to known bladder carcinogens.

Rarer tumours

The squamous and adenocarcinomas of the bladder are in general treated in the same way as the transitional cell tumours. Generally their prognosis is worse and they respond less well to non-surgical treatments.

Testis

Epidemiology

Testicular tumours occur most commonly in men aged between 20 and 40. In the UK there are just over 1000 cases per year which is five times the incidence in Japan. In the US it is more common in white people than in black people.

Aetiology

Many testicular tumours are thought to arise as a developmental abnormality in those with maldescent which increases the likelihood of a testicular tumour by up to 40-fold. Other factors are a contralateral testicular tumour (the incidence of second malignancy in the other testis being around 3 per cent) and possibly previous orchitis, although this remains speculative.

Pathology

There are two main types of testicular tumour: seminoma and teratoma. Around 40 per cent are seminomas and 32 per cent teratomas with a further 14 per cent which contain components of both seminoma and teratoma.

Macroscopically seminomas are solid tumours, well circumscribed, often lobulated and pale in appearance. In contrast teratomas are often haemorrhagic and contain cystic areas.

Microscopically seminoma is composed of sheets of uniform rounded cells and may contain granulomata. Particularly well-differentiated variants are recognized (spermatocytic seminoma) as are more aggressive types (anaplastic seminoma).

In contrast teratoma may contain a range of cell types with varying differentiation. Undifferentiated teratoma contains no recognizable mature elements. Trophoblastic elements may predominate and there may be recognizable yolk sac elements.

Natural history

Testicular tumours invade locally into the tunica vaginalis and along the spermatic cord.

Lymph node spread occurs relatively early to para-aortic nodes and thence to mediastinal nodes.

Blood-borne spread is most commonly to the lungs and liver.

Symptoms

- Testicular swelling or discomfort, particularly with a past history of maldescent.
- Back ache from enlarged para-aortic nodes.
- Cough, haemoptysis or dyspnoea from lung metastases.

Signs

- Testicular swelling which may have an associated hydrocele.
- Central abdominal mass due to palpable nodes.
- Pleural effusion.

Differential diagnosis

- Benign hydrocele.
- Testicular torsion.
- Other causes of backache such as degenerative spinal disease.
- Other causes of lymphadenopathy, e.g. lymphoma.

Investigations

Routine investigations may demonstrate renal impairment due to ureteric obstruction by enlarged para-aortic nodes. Abnormal liver function tests may reflect liver metastases. Chest X-ray may demonstrate metastases as either lung deposits or pleural effusion.

There are specific serum markers for germ cell tumours. These are serum α-foetoprotein (AFP) and β human chorionic gonadotrophin (HCG) and should be measured both prior to any surgical intervention and serially thereafter. Placental alkaline phosphatase is of value for seminoma but is also affected by cigarette smoking and may therefore be misleading in smokers. Around 90 per cent of patients with teratoma will have either AFP or HCG elevated and 40–50 per cent will have both markers raised. The absolute level and rate of fall after treatment are useful prognostic features.

CT scanning of the pelvis and abdomen is essential to evaluate pelvic nodes and liver and CT scanning of the lungs will give accurate assessment of lung metastases.

Staging

The TNM staging system is sometimes used to describe the extent of the primary tumour but for the overall disease the Royal Marsden Hospital staging system is more widely applied. This is shown in Table 10.4.

Treatment

All patients will proceed to inguinal orchidectomy with removal of the affected testis. Scrotal interference should be avoided at all costs because of the risk of tumour implantation in the scrotal wound and subsequent relapse.

Stage 1 tumours

Where after extensive staging there is no evidence of residual tumour after surgery then the prognosis is extremely good and around 85 per cent of patients will be cured with no further treatment.

Seminomas proceed to a course of radiotherapy to the para-aortic nodes. Conventionally the ipsilateral pelvic nodes are also included although this may not be necessary. A low dose of only 30 Gy is required.

Teratomas are entered into a programme of intensive surveillance with monthly measurement of serum markers and regular abdominal and chest CT scans. Those with adverse features such as anaplastic tumour and vascular invasion will receive a short course of chemotherapy.

Stage 2, 3 or 4 tumours

Seminomas will proceed to chemotherapy for all but those with very small para-aortic nodes (stage 2A). The drugs used are usually cisplatin or carboplatin with the possible addition of etoposide. Small volume disease may be treated by radiotherapy alone to the para-aortic and pelvic nodes and radiotherapy will often be given following chemotherapy in other patients.

Teratomas will proceed to chemotherapy. For good prognosis tumours standard chemotherapy will be 3-weekly cycles of BEP (bleomycin, etoposide and cisplatin). High risk patients with extensive disease or very high markers (AFP > 1000, HCG > 10 000) will receive more intensive regimes using weekly administration of alternating drug schedules containing bleomycin, vincristine, cisplatin, methotrexate and etoposide (BOP or POMBACE).

Tumour-related complications

- Gynaecomastia due to high levels of HCG.

Table 10.4 Staging of testicular cancer

T stage		Royal Marsden stage
T1 limited to testis	I	limited to testis
T2 involving tunica albuginea or epididymis	II	involving nodes below diaphragm
T3 invading spermatic cord	III	involving nodes both sides of diaphragm
T4 invading scrotum	IV	distant metastases IVL lungs IVH liver
N1 single node = or < 2 cm max diameter		
N2 single node 2 to 5 cm max diameter or multiple nodes < 5 cm max diameter		
N3 any node > 5 cm max diameter		
M1 distant metastases		

Treatment-related complications

- Unilateral orchidectomy has no physiological effect on potency.
- Abdominal radiotherapy may be related to subsequent peptic ulceration.
- Chemotherapy causes alopecia which is reversible.
- Bleomycin may cause skin changes and pneumonitis in high dose.
- Fertility is impaired after chemotherapy but there are increasing reports of success in fathering children after treatment for testicular cancer. Potency is not affected.

Prognosis

Few patients die from testicular cancer today. Cure is virtually guaranteed for stage 1 tumours and is expected in around 85 per cent of those with more advanced stages.

Screening

Health education programmes aimed at self-examination are the main form of population screening

Rarer tumours

The remaining tumours that occur in the testis are lymphomas (7 per cent) and the rare pure yolk sac tumours, Sertoli cell tumours and interstitial cell tumours. Mesotheliomas arising from the tunica vaginalis are also described. Lymphomas are managed as for any extranodal lymphoma while other rare tumours are managed by surgical excision.

Penis

Epidemiology

Penile cancer is rare in this country with only 300 cases reported per year, and it accounts for less than 1 per cent of deaths from cancer in men. It is more common in other parts of the world, in particular Africa and China where it accounts for around 15 per cent of male cancers.

Aetiology

It is virtually unknown in populations who practice circumcision. A relationship with papilloma virus has also been proposed.

Pathology

Macroscopically it may be a papilliferous or solid growth on the shaft or glans of the penis. Ulceration may occur. It may develop insidiously beneath the foreskin.

Microscopically penile cancer is a squamous carcinoma often well or moderately differentiated.

Natural history

The tumour will invade the shaft of the penis and spread to inguinal lymph nodes, as shown in Figure 10.3. Blood-borne spread occurs relatively late to lungs and liver.

Symptoms

Tumours are usually asymptomatic other than local discharge and odour.

Signs

The primary tumour is usually obvious on clinical examination. Palpable inguinal nodes are present in up to half of patients.

Differential diagnosis

Other penile skin lesions should be considered, including lympho-granuloma venereum, condylomata acuminata, chancroid, traumatic ulceration, leukoplakia, Bowen's disease, erythroplasia of Queyrat and giant penile condylomata (Buschke–Lowenstein tumour).

Other causes of inguinal lymphadenopathy need to be taken into account, in particular chronic infection which accounts for around 50 per cent of the associated lymphadenopathy.

Investigations

Routine investigations are rarely helpful although a chest X-ray will be necessary to exclude lung metastases.

Fig. 10.3 Advanced right inguinal node disease due to metastases from a carcinoma of the penis. The primary tumour was treated some months earlier when no metastases were apparent by penile amputation.

A biopsy or cytological scrapings will confirm the diagnosis.

Fine needle aspiration of enlarged nodes should be used to distinguish metastatic nodes from infected and inflammatory nodes.

Where inguinal nodes are involved a pelvic CT scan is of value to assess further lymphatic spread.

Staging

The commonly used staging system is the Jackson staging which is shown alongside the formal TNM staging in Table 10.5.

Treatment

Radical treatment

This will be appropriate even where there is inguinal node involvement.

Surgery

This will involve partial or complete amputation as shown in Figure 10.3.

Radical radiotherapy

This can be delivered by either external beam treatment or the use of a penile mould. The penis is preserved and this is usually therefore the initial treatment of choice reserving surgery for salvage.

Treatment of involved nodes should be by block dissection of the groin. In the case of fixed inoperable nodes then local irradiation can be performed. Advanced fixed fungating nodes are shown in Figure 10.3.

Palliative treatment

This may be indicated for locally advanced disease or where there are distant metastases. Usually a short palliative course of radiotherapy to the primary site, nodes or local recurrence will help prevent local pain and fungation.

There is no recognized chemotherapy for penile cancer although responses are seen in advanced disease using schedules containing drugs such as cisplatinum, methotrexate, 5-flurouracil and mitomycin C.

Table 10.5   Staging for cancer of the penis

T stage	Jackson stage	
T1 superficial subepithelial	I	limited to glans or prepuce
T2 invading corpus cavernosa	II	invading shaft; no nodes
T3 invading urethra or prostate	III	invading shaft; node positive
T4 invading adjacent structures	IV	fixed inoperable nodes or distant metastases

Tumour-related complications

Interference with micturition and potency is seen.

Treatment-related complications

Radiotherapy may result in urethral stricture in about 10 per cent of cases.

Prognosis

Survival with stage 1 disease is over 85 per cent at 5 years falling to 35 per cent for stage 3 tumours. Long-term survival with stage 4 disease is unusual.

11

Gynaecological cancer

Cervix

Epidemiology

Carcinoma of the cervix accounts for around 20 per cent of cancers in women, being third in order of incidence after breast and lung cancer, with around 4500 cases each year in the UK. It is predominantly a disease a women in their 40s and 50s but is showing an increase in younger age groups. It is common in lower socio-economic groups and there is a wide geographical variation, highest levels of the disease being in South America with incidence figures of up to 80 in 100 000 compared to 12 in 100 000 in the UK.

Aetiology

Associated with sexual activity, being increased in women starting inter-course at an early age and having multiple partners. It is more common in women who are or who have been married than in single women. There is some evidence that the male partner is implicated, being associated with partners of lower socio-economic groups and the identification of high risk males who have more than one partner who develops cervical cancer.

Viral with both herpes simplex type 2 infection and human papilloma virus types 16 and 18 being implicated.

Pathology

Macroscopically there are two common presentations:

1. Proliferative growth at the cervix with surface ulceration.
2. Diffusely infiltrating tumour with the mucosa intact due to tumour arising in the endocervical canal. The latter is sometimes described as a barrel-cervix.

Microscopically 95 per cent of cervical cancers are squamous carcino-mas of varying differentiation. The remaining 5 per cent are adenocarci-nomas arising from the external os or endocervix.

Natural history

Local spread in all directions occurs as shown in Figure 11.1.

Lymph node spread occurs relatively early, being identified in around 15 per cent of stage 1 tumours. From paracervical nodes there is spread to internal and external iliac nodes, presacral and obturator nodes. Subsequent spread is then up the para-aortic node chain.

Blood-borne metastases occur affecting in particular the lungs, liver and bone.

Symptoms

- Asymptomatic presentation as a result of an abnormal cervical smear.
- Vaginal bleeding particularly after intercourse.
- Vaginal discharge.
- Local pain is unusual unless there is extensive pelvic infiltration.
- Renal failure is a recognized presentation due to bilateral ureteric obstruction.
- Other symptoms of local spread may include haematuria or rectal bleeding.

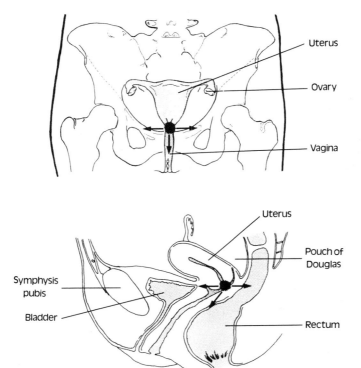

Fig. 11.1 Patterns of spread from carcinoma of the cervix.

- Pelvic and para-aortic lymphadenopathy may cause low back and sacral pain.
- General symptoms of malignancy including anorexia, malaise and weight loss may also be present.

Signs

Pelvic examination is mandatory at which the tumour will usually be apparent at the cervix as a proliferative or ulcerative growth or a diffuse infiltration. It is important to note extension onto the vaginal mucosa and on rectal examination any evidence of spread into the parametrium or rectal mucosa.

Differential diagnosis

Other cervical lesions should be considered, such as a cervical erosion.

Where bladder or rectal involvement is diagnosed it may be difficult to distinguish clinically between primary tumours of these sites invading the cervix although this is usually apparent on histology.

Investigations

Routine investigations may reveal anaemia due to bleeding and a raised white cell count where there has been chronic infection. Renal failure will be apparent on routine biochemical tests and a chest X-ray will be needed to exclude metastases.

Cervical cytology may have been performed to diagnose malignancy and vaginal swabs may demonstrate the nature of an infective discharge.

A full examination under anaesthetic including a cystoscopy should be performed in all cases at which time biopsies can also be taken.

A CT scan of the abdomen and pelvis will help assess local extension and enlargement of pelvic and para-aortic lymph nodes.

An IVU will assess ureteric obstruction although this can now usually be seen clearly on CT.

A bipedal lymphangiogram has been used in the past to visualize pelvic and para-aortic lymph nodes. This may supplement information from CT but in practice the two investigations are not usually performed and in most centres CT will be the imaging of first choice.

Staging

The FIGO staging system is generally accepted in clinical assessment of cervical cancer, as shown in Table 11.1.

Treatment

Radical treatment will be considered for all patients except those with widespread metastatic disease or bladder or rectal involvement. Presentation with renal failure is not an absolute contraindication to radical treatment and in selected cases percutaneous nephrostomies to re-establish renal drainage may be performed prior to treatment.

Localized to the cervix (stage 1)

Surgery

Radical surgery is the treatment of choice in the form of a radical hysterectomy (Wertheim's hysterectomy) during which, in addition to the removal of the uterus tubes and ovaries, the upper vagina, parametrium and pelvic lymph nodes are also included in the resection.

Radiotherapy

Radical radiotherapy may be given for early stage cancer of the cervix and the results in terms of survival are no worse than those after radical surgery although there may be a greater incidence of long-term morbidity. It is usually therefore reserved for elderly patients and those medically unfit for surgery but is an acceptable option for younger women who refuse surgery.

Post-operative radiotherapy may be indicated following Wertheim's hysterectomy where the excision margins are not clear of tumour and where there is involvement of the removed pelvic lymph nodes in the resection.

Pre-operative radiotherapy has been advocated in the past but it has no proven value and using the above criteria only 20 per cent of women will require irradiation in addition to surgery.

Tumour beyond cervix (stages 2 and 3)

Radiotherapy

Radical radiotherapy will be the treatment of choice. This will involve a course of external beam treatment to the whole pelvis covering the major node chains up to the bifurcation of the aorta delivering a dose of 40 to

Table 11.1 FIGO staging for cancer of the cervix

Stage 1	
(a)	Microinvasive disease limited to the cervix
(b)	Confined to the cervix with invasion > 5 mm depth from surface
Stage 2	
(a)	Extension to vaginal mucosa but not into lower third of vagina
(b)	Extension to parametrium but not reaching pelvic side wall
Stage 3	
(a)	Extension to lower third of vagina
(b)	Extension to pelvic side wall
Stage 4	
(a)	Involvement of bladder or rectal mucosa
(b)	Distant metastases

50 Gy over 4 to 5 weeks. Intracavitary treatment to the cervix will follow this using an intrauterine tube and vaginal source to give a further 25 to 30 Gy to the cervix and surrounding tissues.

Palliation

Where there are distant metastases or locally advanced pelvic disease then radical local treatment is inappropriate. Chemotherapy for advanced and recurrent disease has only limited activity and complete response is extremely rare. The most effective drug schedules are combinations of cisplatin, methotrexate and ifosfamide and there may be considerable associated toxicity.

Palliative radiotherapy for advanced local disease may be worthwhile and is particularly indicated for the control of local bleeding and pelvic pain. Other procedures such as a palliative colostomy may be required where there is rectal involvement or fistulae form.

Hormone replacement

Cervical cancer is not hormone dependent. This means that hormone manipulation is not a useful approach to treatment but also that following radical treatment, in young women particularly, hormone replacement therapy should be considered.

Tumour-related complications

- Renal failure due to bilateral ureteric obstruction.
- Fistulae between bladder or rectum and vagina.
- Pyometra due to obstruction of the cervical canal by tumour.

Treatment-related complications

Radical surgery may result in urinary urgency and urge or stress incontinence.

Radical radiotherapy may result acutely in bowel and bladder toxicity with a radiation cystitis and diarrhoea.

Long-term sequelae from radiotherapy may include reduced bladder volume, telangiectasia causing haematuria or rectal bleeding, chronic diarrhoea and vaginal stenosis. Rarely bowel or bladder fistulae may occur although subsequent investigations often reveal recurrent disease in this setting.

Prognosis

Outcome is closely related to stage at presentation with a 5 year survival of around 80 per cent for stage 1 and 2A tumours falling to only 20–30 per cent for stage 3 and less than 5 per cent for stage 4. Within stage 1 tumours prognosis is related to tumour bulk and differentiation.

For microinvasive and *in situ* carcinoma of the cervix surgery is almost always curative emphasizing the importance of early diagnosis in this condition where curative treatment is readily available for early stage disease.

Screening

Screening for cervical neoplasia by cervical smear testing is widespread and there is good evidence that in the US and Scandinavia the rate of decline in cervical cancer can be related to intensity of screening. Currently around 3 million cervical smears are performed in Britain each year and it has been estimated that this has reduced the incidence of invasive cancers by around 30 per cent. Current recommendations are for all sexually active women below the age of 50 years to have cervical smears at 3 to 5 yearly intervals. A major problem with this as with any screening programme is to achieve good rates of compliance particularly in those groups at high risk.

Future prospects

The greatest impact is likely to be made by extending the current screening programmes to reach all those women at risk with high rates of compliance in order to detect early curable disease.

Current developments in treatment are looking at the role of adjuvant chemotherapy in the radical treatment of cervical cancer and the possible role of biological modifying agents in the treatment of more advanced disease.

Rarer tumours

Five per cent of cervical cancers are adenocarcinomas. These are generally treated in the same way as the more common squamous cancers and, stage for stage, they have a similar prognosis.

Endometrium

Epidemiology

Compared to cancer of the cervix, cancer of the endometrium affects the older, predominantly post-menopausal age group. The incidence in the UK is similar to that of cervical cancer with around 4000 cases each year, although the mortality is lower which reflects its natural history. There is far less geographical variation than cervical cancer although it is relatively rare in Japan where the incidence is about one-tenth of that in Europe and the US.

Aetiology

Endometrial carcinoma occurs typically in obese nulliparous women who have a tendency to diabetes and cardiovascular disease.

High levels of circulating oestrogens are a known cause and it is a recognized complication of an oestrogen-secreting granulosa cell tumour of the ovary. There is no proven association with therapeutic use of oestrogens in hormone replacement therapy and despite isolated reports an association with prolonged tamoxifen use for breast cancer has yet to be substantiated.

Pathology

Macroscopically the tumour arises within the uterine cavity and may be polypoid or a more diffuse even multifocal growth arising from the endometrium.

Microscopically the tumour is an adenocarcinoma which may be of varying grade, usually designated from G1 (well differentiated) to G3 (poorly differentiated).

Natural history

There is local invasion into the myometrium and cervix. The tubes and ovaries may also be involved and the tumour occasionally extends into parametrial tissues or involves the bladder or rectum. This is far less common than in cancer of the cervix.

Lymph node spread may occur involving pelvic lymph nodes, and submucosal lymphatic permeation along the vaginal walls is well recognized.

Distant metastases by blood-borne spread most frequently involves lungs and bone.

Symptoms

The classic presentation of endometrial cancer is with post-menopausal bleeding. In the pre-menopausal woman heavy and/or irregular periods may be the only symptom. There may be an associated vaginal discharge.

General symptoms of malaise, anorexia and weight loss are usually mild and symptoms from metastatic disease are unusual at presentation.

Signs

On pelvic examination the uterus may feel bulky and a vaginal discharge or bleeding from the os may be apparent. Often no physical signs can be detected.

Differential diagnosis

Other causes of post-menopausal bleeding should be considered such as atrophic vaginitis and in pre-menopausal women other causes of irregular menstrual bleeding such as fibroids.

Investigations

Routine investigations may reveal anaemia due to chronic blood loss. Other abnormalities are unusual.

The diagnosis is made by examination under anaesthetic at which time the cervical canal and uterine cavity are dilated in turn and fractional curettage performed to obtain endometrial samples.

A chest X-ray will be performed to exclude distant metastases.

Further imaging of the pelvis is usually reserved for more advanced cases (stage 2, 3 or 4) when a CT scan will be used to assess local spread and lymph node status.

Staging

Carcinoma of the endometrium is staged using the FIGO system, as shown in Table 11.2.

Treatment

A major feature of endometrial cancer is the predominance of stage 1 tumours at presentation accounting for 70–80 per cent of patients.

Surgery

Total abdominal hysterectomy and bilateral salpingo-oophorectomy is the treatment of choice for disease localized to the endometrium.

A Wertheim's hysterectomy (see above) is indicated when there is cervical involvement (stage 2).

Radiotherapy

Post-operative radiotherapy is given to patients following hysterectomy for stage 1 disease depending on the risk factors for local and distant dissemination. Well-differentiated tumours with minimal myometrial invasion will receive vaginal irradiation only; moderately or poorly differentiated tumours and those invading into the mid or outer third of the myometrium are considered to have a greater risk of lymph node spread and therefore receive both external beam radiotherapy to the pelvic nodes and intra-

Table 11.2   FIGO staging for cancer of the endometrium

Stage 1	
(a)	Confined to the endometrium; no myometrial invasion
(b)	Confined to the endometrium; invasion < 50% of myometrium
(c)	Confined to the endometrium; invasion > 50% of myometrium
Stage 2	Invasion of cervix
Stage 3	Spread to pelvic tissues
Stage 4	
(a)	Spread to bladder or rectum
(b)	Distant metastases

vaginal treatment.

Radical radiotherapy may on occasions be given for elderly unfit patients with stage 1 disease and those with bulky stage 2 and stage 3 tumours. This will take the form of external beam treatment to the pelvis followed by intracavitary treatment to the uterine cavity and upper vagina.

Palliative treatment

Palliative radiotherapy may be given for locally advanced tumours and for painful bone metastases.

Endometrial cancer is a hormone-dependent tumour and metastatic disease will respond to progestogens such as medroxyprogesterone acetate or megestrol. Response rates are between 20 and 30 per cent and useful palliation of symptomatic metastases may be achieved. Responses to gonadotrophin-releasing hormone analogues such as leuprorelin are also recognized. There is no good evidence to support the use of these agents as adjuvant treatment, although they are sometimes given in this setting.

Tumour-related complications

Pyometra or haematometra may occur due to obstruction of the uterine cavity.

Treatment-related complications

Hysterectomy may result in urinary urgency and urge or stress incontinence.

Pelvic radiotherapy may be associated with late bowel and bladder toxicity causing frequency, haematuria, and rectal bleeding, rectal and vaginal stenosis.

Prognosis

The prognosis for endometrial carcinoma is good since the majority of patients present with stage 1 disease for which there are cure rates in excess of 85 per cent. Prognosis for more advanced stages falls as would be anticipated with 5 year survival rates of around 65 per cent for stage 2 and 35 per cent for stage 3.

Prevention

The early diagnosis of endometrial cancer is aided by its early presentation with post-menopausal bleeding. It is therefore vital that all women with this symptom are investigated appropriately to exclude endometrial cancer.

Rarer tumours

Sarcomas of the endometrium may arise presenting in the same way as endometrial cancer. They may be pure sarcomas such as a leiomyosarcoma arising from a fibroid or mixed tumours such as the mixed mesodermal tumour which contains both epithelial and stromal components, the latter in the form of malignant sarcomatous cells.

The prognosis for endometrial sarcomas is poor. Treatment is surgical removal at hysterectomy and post-operative radiotherapy is usually given to reduce the likelihood of local relapse. There is no proven role for chemotherapy although distant metastases are a common problem with these tumours.

Ovary

Epidemiology

There are around 5000 cases of carcinoma of the ovary in the UK each year, accounting for around 5 per cent of cancer in women and 4000 deaths per year. There is a similar incidence in the US but a low incidence in Japan which approaches that of American women in immigrants to the US.

Aetiology

Ovarian cancer tends to occur in women over the age of 40 years who are nulliparous and of higher socio-economic groups. There is an association with blood group A.

No specific environmental agents have been identified as directly contributing to the development of ovarian cancer.

A familial pattern is seen in some cases.

Pathology

The common appearance of ovarian cancer is that of a cystic enlargement of the ovary. Two common types are recognized macroscopically:

1. The pseudomucinous cyst characteristically being a large multiloculated tumour mass containing mucinous material.
2. The serous cyst containing clear fluid within a thin-walled cyst containing papillary structures.

Other tumours may form solid masses (typical of a Brenner tumour) or characteristic teratomas.

The microscopic appearances of ovarian cancer are variable and the classification often complex.

Epithelial adenocarcinomas are the common ovarian cancers with several variants recognized such as clear cell carcinomas and endometrioid carcinomas. Germ cell tumours are the other major group of tumours of the ovary but in contrast to the testis the majority are benign teratomas.

Rarer tumours include those derived from gonadal stroma such as the granulosa cell and Sertoli cell tumours which are oestrogen and androgen secreting respectively, and mixed mesodermal tumours analogous to those which grow in the uterus and lymphomas.

Metastases may also present in the ovary, typically from carcinoma of the breast or stomach (Krukenberg tumours).

Natural history

Local growth occurs within the ovary spreading through a cyst wall onto the surface.

Transcoelomic spread across the peritoneal cavity results in the classical appearance of multiple seedlings visible throughout the pelvic and abdominal cavities studding the peritoneal surfaces. Involvement of the omentum is also common and ascites is frequently found at operation.

Lymph node spread occurs to para-aortic nodes in the first instance.

Blood-borne metastases to liver and lungs are seen in more advanced disease.

Meig's syndrome is the presence of a pleural effusion accompanying an ovarian tumour which has the features of a transudate and is cytologically negative for carcinoma cells.

Symptoms

Ovarian cancer may remain asymptomatic for some time and often presents with vague symptoms of abdominal discomfort and pelvic pain. In more advanced cases this may be associated with abdominal swelling due to either tumour or ascites and urinary and bowel disturbance due to local pressure.

General symptoms of malignancy including malaise, anorexia and weight loss may also be present and metastases may cause dyspnoea or bone pain.

Signs

Abdominal swelling and distension with a palpable mass or clinical signs of free fluid (shifting dullness to percussion and a fluid thrill) may be present.

An ovarian mass may be palpable per vaginam or per rectum.

A pleural effusion may be detectable clinically by dullness to percussion and absent breath sounds.

A left supraclavicular node may be palpable in advanced cases.

Differential diagnosis

Other causes of abdominal swelling should be considered including ascites from other causes, hepatomegaly or splenomegaly, benign ovarian masses and intestinal obstruction.

Investigations

Routine investigations will often be unremarkable although in advanced cases there may be electrolyte disturbance from intestinal obstruction or ureteric obstruction causing renal failure. Chest X-ray may demonstrate metastases or a pleural effusion.

Ultrasound will image the ovaries and give information regarding the nature of ovarian cysts. Liver ultrasound will evaluate the presence or absence of liver metastases

CT scan of the abdomen and pelvis will demonstrate the primary tumour and also pelvic and para-aortic lymph node enlargement together with liver metastases if present. An example of a massive intra-abdominal tumour mass from carcinoma of the ovary is shown in Figure 11.2.

Serum CA125 is a valuable blood marker for ovarian cancer and is a useful monitor of response to treatment.

Creatinine clearance or EDTA clearance may be necessary for those patients requiring chemotherapy.

Staging

The FIGO staging system for ovarian cancer is in common use, as shown in Table 11.3.

Treatment

Surgery

All patients with operable disease will proceed to laparotomy at which total abdominal hysterectomy, bilateral salpingo-oophorectomy and omentectomy are performed together with careful examination of the para-aortic nodes, liver and peritoneal surfaces including the subdiaphragmatic regions and biopsy of any suspicious areas. Prognosis is directly related to the residual bulk of tumour and so maximum tumour debulking should be attempted in all patients even where complete clearance is not possible.

Fig. 11.2 CT scan showing extensive intra-abdominal tumour from carcinoma of the ovary.

For patients with stage 1 disease who have a normal post-operative CT scan and normal CA125 levels no further treatment is indicated and close observation with serial CT scans or pelvic ultrasounds and serum CA125 levels will be done.

Chemotherapy

For more advanced disease localized to the abdominopelvic cavity, i.e. stages 2 and 3, chemotherapy is indicated. The drug of choice is cisplatin or its analogue carboplatin given for 6 cycles at monthly intervals. There may be a slightly better rate of response for combination therapy adding cyclophosphamide and adriamycin to the drug regime but this will be associated with a corresponding increase in toxicity.

For stage 4 disease with soft tissue metastases the outlook is poor and treatment often not indicated. For patients with good general status chemotherapy may be considered as for earlier stage disease.

Palliative treatment

Chemotherapy may be of value where relapse occurs after a long period of remission (> 1 year). Relapse within the first year rarely responds to further chemotherapy.

Radiotherapy may be of value for symptomatic pelvic masses, vaginal bleeding from disease invading the vagina and bone metastases.

Tumour-related complications

- Ascites and pleural effusions may occur.
- Intestinal obstruction is common in the advanced phases of the disease.

Treatment-related complications

Cisplatin may cause neurotoxicity with peripheral neuropathy or less frequently spinal cord damage. Ototoxicity may result in tinnitus and high tone deafness. Reduced renal function is common but overt renal failure should not occur provided the patient is well hydrated and renal function is properly monitored.

Carboplatin may cause significant bone marrow depression.

Table 11.3   FIGO staging for cancer of the ovary

Stage 1	Confined to the ovary
(a)	One ovary involved
(b)	both ovaries involved
Stage 2	Spread to the pelvis
Stage 3	Spread to the abdominal cavity
Stage 4	Blood-borne metastases

Prognosis

The outlook for stage 1 ovarian cancer is good with 10 year survival figures of over 80 per cent. For more advanced disease the results of current chemotherapy give 5 year survival figures of 35–50 per cent. The survival of patients with stage 4 disease is usually only a few months.

Screening

Screening programmes for ovarian cancer have been proposed using serum CA125 measurements and abdominal ultrasound. Currently they are recommended for those with a strong positive family history but routine population screening is not justified.

Rare tumours

Brenner tumours

Fibromas of the ovary, usually benign in nature. Treatment is surgical removal.

Teratomas

Arising in the ovary these are usually benign although malignant teratomas analogous to those arising in the testis are recognized. Treatment should include adjuvant chemotherapy following surgical removal using drug combinations such as BEP (bleomycin, etoposide and cisplatin).

Dysgerminomas

Germ cell tumours arising in the ovary analogous to seminomas arising in the testis. For stage 1 tumours surgery is often curative. More advanced tumours are usually very radiosensitive and post-operative pelvic radiotherapy is recommended. Chemotherapy using drugs such as VAC (vincristine, actinomycin D and cyclophosphamide) may be used for more widespread disease.

Granulosa cell tumours

Granulosa cell tumours are usually of a low grade and generally cured by surgery although local recurrence some years later is recognized. Characteristically they secrete oestrogens and may be associated with the synchronous development of an endometrial cancer.

Sertoli–Leydig cell tumours

Sertoli–Leydig cell tumours are usually of low malignant potential and cured by oophorectomy.

Sarcomas

Rare and typically mixed mesodermal tumours having both sarcomatous and epithelial elements. Their prognosis is poor unless localized within the ovary at the time of surgery.

Lymphomas

May arise within the ovary and are typically high grade non-Hodgkin's lymphomas treated as extra nodal lymphomas at any other site with adjuvant chemotherapy with or without pelvic radiotherapy.

Metastases

May present in the ovary usually from stomach or breast cancer. The classic bilateral ovarian metastases from carcinoma of the stomach are sometimes referred to as Krukenberg tumours.

Vagina

Epidemiology

Carcinoma of the vagina is rare accounting for only 1 per cent of all gynaecological cancer and around 130 deaths each year. It is a disease predominantly of elderly women unless associated with maternal use of stilboestrol.

Aetiology

Chronic irritation of the vaginal mucosa is typically seen following long-term use of a vaginal ring pessary for vaginal prolapse.

Stilboestrol: clear cell carcinoma of the vagina may follow maternal use of stilboestrol during pregnancy with tumours developing during adolescence. Vaginal intraepithelial neoplasia (VAIN) is a recognized epithelial change analogous to CIN at the cervix and may progress to frank carcinoma.

Pathology

Macroscopically the tumour may present as an ulcer, papilliferous growth or diffuse infiltration of the vaginal mucosa.

Microscopically the usual picture is of a squamous carcinoma. Rarely, adenocarcinomas may arise and there is the clear cell variant related to stilboestrol.

Natural history

Direct extension results in invasion of the parametrium, bladder or rectum.

Lymph node spread is to internal iliac and pelvic nodes (from the upper two-thirds of the vagina) and to inguinal and femoral nodes (from the lower third).

Blood-borne spread to liver and lungs may also occur in advanced disease.

Symptoms

- Vaginal discharge and bleeding.
- Local pain is unusual unless there has been extensive pelvic infiltration.

Signs

- Tumour will usually be visible on speculum examination.
- Inguinal nodes may be palpable with tumours of the lower vagina.

Differential diagnosis

- Chronic vaginitis.
- Metastases from the cervix or endometrium.
- Tumours of the urethra or Bartholin's gland.

Investigations

The diagnosis will be confirmed at examination under anaesthetic when biopsies can be taken.

Routine investigations may show chronic anaemia from blood loss, and rarely renal failure due to ureteric obstruction from pelvic infiltration or lung metastases on chest X-ray.

Palpable inguinal nodes should be investigated further by fine needle aspiration to distinguish inflammatory nodes from metastases.

Staging should include CT scan of the pelvis to assess pelvic lymph nodes.

Staging

Vaginal carcinoma is staged using the FIGO classification shown in Table 11.4.

Table 11.4 FIGO staging of vaginal cancer

Stage 1	Limited to the vaginal mucosa
Stage 2	Extension to submucosa and parametrium but not to pelvic side walls
Stage 3	Extension to pelvic side wall
Stage 4	Bladder, rectum or distant metastases.

Treatment

Surgery

Early disease in young, fit women is best treated by radical hysterectomy and total vaginectomy with pelvic lymphadenectomy. Inguinal node dissection may also be required for tumours in the lower third of the vagina.

Radiotherapy

Indicated for both early tumours in those unfit for surgery and stage 2 and 3 disease. This will take the form of external beam irradiation to the pelvis including the inguinal nodes for lower third tumours followed by intracavitary treatment to give a high dose of irradiation directly to the vaginal mucosa and immediate tissues.

Palliative treatment

Radiotherapy is helpful for locally advanced or recurrent disease. This may take the form of external beam treatment where there is a major pelvic component or intracavitary teatment for bleeding or ulcerated disease locally in the vagina.

There is no recognized effective chemotherapy for vaginal carcinoma.

Tumour-related complications

- Vaginal haemorrhage and sepsis.
- Renal failure due to urethral obstruction.

Treatment-related complications

- Recognized acute complications of pelvic radiotherapy including radiation cystitis and diarrhoea.
- Late complications may include vaginal stenosis and fistulae into bladder or rectum, particularly where there has been local infiltration by tumour.

Prognosis

Over 80 per cent of stage 1 patients can expect cure; 50 per cent of patients with stage 2 and 30 per cent of those with stage 3 tumours will survive 5 years.

Screening

Female offspring of mothers who received stilboestrol during pregnancy are at recognized high risk and will benefit from regular screening by clinical examination and vaginal smears.

VAIN seems to be related to earlier cervical malignancy and therefore these patients should also receive regular vaginal smears following treatment of a cervical cancer.

Rarer tumours

Adenocarcinoma and clear cell carcinoma are usually treated surgically, reserving radiotherapy for palliation of advanced tumours.

Vulva

Epidemiology

Cancer of the vulva accounts for only 5 per cent of all gynaecological cancers and around 600 cases occur in the UK each year. It is usually seen in older, post-menopausal women.

Aetiology

Chemical carcinogenesis was seen historically in the 'mulespinners' exposed to mineral oils.

There are also dystrophic conditions of the vulval skin including leukoplakia, lichen sclerosus et atrophicus and Paget's disease of the vulva. True carcinoma *in situ* is also seen in the vulval skin.

Pathology

Macroscopically the tumour is typically a papilliferous growth or an ulcer arising from the medial side of the labium majorum. Bilateral tumours may be seen – the so-called 'kissing cancer'.

Microscopically vulval carcinomas are squamous carcinomas. Other rare tumours which can arise in the vulva include basal cell carcinomas, melanomas, sarcomas and tumours of the female urethra and Bartholin's gland.

Natural history

Local invasion of surrounding soft tissue occurs early and in advanced cases pubic bone may become involved.

Lymphatic spread is to the inguinal nodes before progressing along the pelvic node chain.

Blood-borne spread to lungs may occur but is a late event.

Symptoms

There may be long-standing symptoms of skin dystrophy with local irritation.

A lump may be obvious to the patient.

Pain is usually a late symptom due to bone invasion.

Swelling of the legs may occur due to inguinal nodes or femoral vein involvement.

Signs

The local tumour will be apparent as an ulcer or papilliferous growth.
Inguinal nodes may be palpable with associated leg oedema.

Differential diagnosis

Vulval dystrophies, as discussed above.
Infective conditions such as condylomata, lymphogranuloma inguinale or lymphogranuloma venereum. In the past tuberculous or syphilitic lesions have also been described in the differential diagnosis but are rarely seen today.

Investigations

The tumour is usually apparent clinically and diagnosis is confirmed by a full examination under anaesthetic and biopsy.
Palpable nodes should be investigated with fine needle aspiration for cytological confirmation of malignancy as many will be only inflammatory.
In the presence of palpable nodes CT scan of the pelvis will assess proximal spread into the iliac node chain.
Chest X-ray will exclude the presence of lung metastases.

Staging

Staging uses the TNM classification, as shown in Table 11.5.

Treatment

Surgery

Wide excision of the vulva (vulvectomy) with bilateral femoral and inguinal node dissection is usually recommended.

Table 11.5   TNM classification for cancer of the vulva

T1	Confined to the vulva 2 cm or less in diameter
T2	Confined to the vulva > 2 cm in diameter
T3	Involving the urethra, vagina, perineum or anus
T4	Invading the rectal or bladder mucosa, urethral mucosa or underlying bone
N0	No nodes palpable
N1	Mobile nodes in either groin, not clinically suspicious of malignancy
N2	Mobile nodes in either groin, clinically suspicious of malignancy
N3	Fixed or ulcerated nodes

Radiotherapy

For inoperable disease radical radiotherapy can be given using both external beam treatment and interstitial implantation of the tumour. A radical dose may be given but acute reactions in this area can be severe and are often dose limiting.

Palliative treatment

Local toilet surgery may be required or, where there is extensive posterior infiltration, a defunctioning colostomy.

Radiotherapy is of value for local pain, discharge and bleeding.

There is no recognized chemotherapy for vulval carcinoma although responses are described following combinations effective against squamous carcinomas such as mitomycin C and 5FU or methotrexate and 5FU.

Tumour-related complications

Local haemorrhage and discharge may occur.

Oedema of either or both legs may develop due to venous or lymphatic obstruction.

Urethral invasion may cause difficulty with micturition and anal invasion may result in faecal incontinence.

Treatment-related complications

Radical surgery may be complicated by delayed wound healing. Leg oedema may occur where there has been extensive dissection of the groins.

Prognosis

Survival is related to the extent of disease at presentation and general condition which in the frail and elderly may preclude radical surgery.

Following radical surgery for localized disease over 80 per cent of patients will survive 5 years. The presence of lymph nodes is a poor prognostic sign reducing 5 year survival to around 40 per cent.

Rare tumours

Basal cell carcinomas

Usually cured by local surgery unless they have invaded deeper structures. They may also be treated by radiotherapy.

Melanomas

Best treated with wide surgical excision. For more advanced local lesions or patients with distant metastases palliative radiotherapy may be of value in obtaining local control.

Sarcomas

These are also best treated by wide surgical excision.

Choriocarcinoma

Epidemiology

Choriocarcinoma is a malignant tumour arising from the placental tissues. It is a rare tumour which occasionally may arise in association with a normal pregnancy but is far more common as a complication of a hydatidiform mole.

The incidence of hydatidiform mole is around 1 in 1000 pregnancies of which 3 per cent will develop into choriocarcinoma. The incidence of choriocarcinoma following term delivery where there is no mole is around 1 in 50 000 pregnancies. There is no recognized geographical variation.

Aetiology

Hydatidiform mole is more common in pregnancies in women under 20 and over 40.

Past history of a mole predisposes to subsequent mole pregnancies.

Pathology

Macroscopically choriocarcinoma arises within the uterus following normal pregnancy, ectopic pregnancy, spontaneous abortion or hydatidiform mole. It is characteristically a haemorrhagic tumour with no detectable placental remnant.

Microscopically the distinction between a benign mole and choriocarcinoma is made by the absence of villi in the choriocarcinoma with areas of necrosis and haemorrhage. The cells of the trophoblast have malignant features with many mitoses and pleomorphic cells with multiple nucleoli.

Natural history

Local invasion involves the uterine wall at an early stage.

Early blood-borne dissemination occurs to lungs, liver and the central nervous system. Other common distant sites involved are skin, bowel and spleen. Bone metastases are rare.

Lymph node metastases are rare.

Symptoms

- Vaginal bleeding within 1 year of pregnancy.
- Abdominal or pelvic discomfort may be present.

Up to one-third of patients may present with symptoms of metastatic disease such as cough, haemoptysis, weight loss, headache or fits.

Signs

The uterus may be enlarged and tender on pelvic examination or a pelvic mass may be palpable.

Chest signs secondary to lung collapse or effusion may be present, the liver may be enlarged and palpable and there may be focal neurological signs associated with brain metastases.

Differential diagnosis

Choriocarcinoma must be distinguished from hydatidiform mole.

Other causes of uterine bleeding such as fibroids and cervical or endometrial carcinoma should be considered.

Investigations

Blood levels of human chorionic gonadotrophin (HCG) are important. This is raised in normal pregnancy but also with hydatidiform mole and choriocarcinoma. It is an important indicator of tumour bulk in choriocarcinoma and an invaluable tumour marker for monitoring treatment.

Ultrasound of the uterus gives a characteristic picture in hydatidiform mole and choriocarcinoma. It can also be used to assess the extent of local invasion through the uterine wall and fallopian tube and ovarian involvement.

CT scan of the chest is used to exclude pulmonary metastases below the size detectable on plain chest X-ray.

CT scan of the brain may be indicated where there are neurological symptoms or signs.

The diagnosis of choriocarcinoma will be confirmed histologically on examination of the uterine contents removed at examination under anaesthetic and suction evacuation.

Staging

There is no recognized staging system for choriocarcinoma. However, a prognostic score has been described by which patients can be divided into those with a good, intermediate and poor prognosis. This uses a number of parameters including age, parity, preceding pregnancies, HCG level, number, site and size of metastases.

Treatment

Because of its rarity and the complex nature of its treatment all patients should be referred to a major centre experienced in the management of choriocarcinoma.

Surgery

Suction evacuation of the uterus is the initial treatment in all cases.

Chemotherapy

Subsequent chemotherapy is based on close monitoring of serum HCG levels. Indications for treatment include:

- Very high levels persisting after evacuation (> 20 000 iu).
- Rising levels of HCG.
- Continued uterine bleeding.
- Metastatic disease.

All the above are signs of active choriocarcinoma.

Low risk patients

Low risk patients who are young with disease restricted to the uterus and vagina or those with lung metastases are treated with methotrexate as a single agent.

Intermediate risk patients

Intermediate risk patients who are over 39 years with localized disease or have spleen or liver metastases receive chemotherapy with actinomycin D, vincristine and etoposide.

High risk patients

Those with metastases in the gastrointestinal tract or liver receive more intensive chemotherapy using etoposide, actinomycin D, methotrexate, vincristine and cyclophosphamide. Multiple drugs are used in this context to prevent resistance emerging in surviving cells.

Because of the high risk of CNS metastases prophylactic treatment with intrathecal methotrexate is also recommended for high risk patients and all those with lung metastases.

Established CNS metastases are treated with dexamethasone and multiple drug chemotherapy as for the high risk group.

Tumour-related complications

Bleeding from the uterus or metastatic sites resulting in gastointestinal, intracerebral or intrapulmonary haemorrhage may be seen.

Respiratory failure may complicate multiple pulmonary metastases or may be precipitated by their treatment due to rapid tumour lysis.

Treatment-related complications

Rapid tumour destruction with chemotherapy of widespread metastases may cause not only respiratory failure but also extensive metabolic disturbance.

Many patients have proceeded after successful treatment to have further pregnancies without complications. There is, however, some concern that oral contraceptive treatment in the immediate period after chemotherapy may provoke further relapse and oral contraception should be avoided for 6 months following completion of chemotherapy.

Prognosis

The outlook for patients with choriocarcinoma is extremely good. It is only those who have high risk disease including those over 40 years with bulky (> 5 cm) metastases, multiple sites or more than a total of eight metastases, brain metastases and very high HCG levels (> 10 000 iu) in whom survival of less than 100 per cent can be anticipated and even in this group over 80 per cent will be cured.

Screening

Routine screening of pregnant women is not indicated but high risk patients who have had previous trophoblastic disease (mole or choriocarcinoma) should have careful monitoring of HCG following delivery.

12

CNS tumours

A discussion of the general principles will be followed by specific examples.

Epidemiology

These are uncommon tumours with 3000 new cases and a similar number of deaths registered in the UK per annum. One to two per cent of autopsies performed after death from other causes reveal occult brain primary tumours. There is a bimodal age incidence with peaks at 5–9 and 50–55 years, varying with the type of tumour, e.g. medulloblastomas are very rare beyond adolescence, glioblastomas are very rare in adolescents and children. There is a slight male predominance in all types except meningioma.

Aetiology

In the vast majority of cases no aetiological factors can be identified. Several associations have been identified but these conditions are themselves very rare:

1. Neurofibromatosis – neurofibroma and neurofibrosarcoma.
2. Tuberose sclerosis – glioma and hamartoma.
3. von Hippel-Lindau syndrome – cerebellar haemangioblastoma.
4. Gorlin's syndrome – medulloblastoma.

Pathology

Classification of tumours according to their cell of origin is outlined in Table 12.1.

Eighty per cent are intracranial and 20 per cent spinal, childhood tumours tending to be located in the cerebellum, adult tumours in the cerebral hemispheres. Highly malignant tumours will have necrosis and haemorrhage on cut section, oedema of the surrounding cerebral tissue, and may not be well circumscribed. Multifocal high grade gliomas and lymphomas are recognized. Calcification is seen in craniopharyngiomas, oligodendrogliomas and some meningiomas, making them visible on a plain skull X-ray.

Table 12.1   Classification of CNS tumours according to the tissue of origin

Gliomas (50%)	Astrocytoma, oligodendroglioma, ependymoma
Meninges (25%)	Meningioma, meningiosarcoma
Pituitary tumours (20%)	Craniopharyngioma, adenoma
Vascular tissue (2%)	Angioma, haemangioblastoma
Pineal tumours (<1%)	Pinealoma, pineoblastoma
Germ cells (<1%)	Teratoma, dysgerminoma
Miscellaneous	Chordoma, medulloblastoma, lymphoma

Spinal tumours may be classified further according to their origin in relation to the dural/spinal cord anatomy:

1. Extradural, e.g. metastases, chordoma.
2. Intradural extramedullary, e.g. meningiomas, neurofibromas.
3. Intramedullary, e.g. astrocytomas, ependymomas, haemangioblastomas, lipomas, dermoids.

Tumours may be subclassified into grades according to the degree of differentiation. This grading reflects the expected behaviour of the tumour and takes into account factors such as the degree of tumour cellularity, the number and appearance of mitotic figures and the presence of necrosis.

Natural history

Direct infiltration is the main mode of spread and the cause of death of the majority of patients dying from CNS tumours. All CNS tumours, even if benign, enlarge by infiltrating and/or compressing the adjacent neural tissue, and in turn the increasing peritumoural oedema leads to raised intracranial pressure. Raised intracranial pressure may also be due to hydrocephalus from compression of the ventricular system leading to impaired drainage of cerebrospinal fluid (CSF) and ventricular dilatation proximal to the block. Local infiltration will also lead to focal brain damage manifested as focal neurological signs, and some tumours cross the corpus callosum in the midline to involve the contralateral hemisphere.

Tumours prone to CSF seeding include medulloblastoma, ependymoma, pineoblastoma, germ cell tumours and lymphoma. This results in meningeal deposits anywhere from the foramen magnum down to the 4th sacral vertebra. Insertion of a shunt to relieve hydrocephalus may rarely lead to distant dissemination of tumour.

Lymphatic spread is not seen as the neural tissue does not have a true lymphatic drainage system.

Distant metastases are extremely rare, but are described in patients with very aggressive tumours such as glioblastomas which have invaded the dural venous sinus system and in medulloblastomas.

Presentation

Cerebral tumours

Patients with cerebral tumours usually present with one or more of the following:

1. Epilepsy – the patient presents with an epileptic fit which may be generalized, affecting the whole body or focal, or affecting a region or single part of the body which is related to the anatomical origin within the brain. A cerebral tumour should be considered in any patient presenting *de novo* in this manner, particularly with focal epilepsy.
2. Raised intracranial pressure – the patient may complain of headaches with an early morning predominance, nausea, vomiting, somnolence, apathy, poor concentration, memory impairment and personality change. Clinically, there may be papilloedema, upgoing plantar responses, evidence of impaired higher mental functions and impairment of consciousness.
3. Focal neurological deficit – local pressure from a tumour will lead to dysfunction of the affected tissue due to ischaemia which will be manifested clinically by focal neurological signs corresponding to the affected portion of the brain. These will be upper motor neurone in type, e.g. spasticity, hyper-reflexia and upgoing plantars in the case of a hemiparesis.

Spinal tumours

These may present with one or more of the following.

Spinal cord compression

This is seen when the lesion lies between the foramen magnum and the lower limit of the cord at the junction of the 1st and 2nd lumbar vertebrae. There will be a pattern of upper motor neurone loss of function below the level of the block, associated with a sensory level and sphincter disturbance.

Cauda equina compression

The lesion will lie somewhere below the lower limit of the spinal cord affecting only nerve roots and therefore the signs are those of a lower motor neurone lesion affecting the lower limbs, i.e. hypotonia, weakness, wasting, fasciculation, hyporeflexia, downgoing plantar reflexes and a dermatomal sensory loss. The urethral and anal sphincters may also be impaired.

Investigations

Cerebral tumours

Contrast enhanced CT scan

This is mandatory to give information regarding the location, size and degree of local invasion of the tumour. Magnetic resonance imaging (MRI) is considered to give greater information in this respect but is less widely available. Isotope brain scans have been superseded and are inferior to a CT scan, particularly with respect to evaluation of posterior fossa tumours.

Stereotactic percutaneous needle biopsy or open biopsy

This is essential to obtain a specimen for histological diagnosis. When surgical resection is not feasible, e.g. a tumour located at a critical site such as the brain stem, a needle biopsy will be the least traumatic means of sampling a tumour. Otherwise open biopsy and tumourectomy are performed, and have the advantages of providing a larger specimen for histological analysis and potentially being of therapeutic benefit.

Lumbar puncture

This may be of value in providing further information to assist in diagnosis and treatment, e.g. in providing CSF for cytology in carcinomatous meningitis and, in the case of germ cell tumours, allowing assay of CSF α foetoprotein and β human chorionic gonadotrophin. However, a lumbar puncture should not be routinely performed in patients with brain tumours due to the risk of coning (compression and herniation of the brain stem through the foramen magnum) which may be fatal and should always be preceded by a CT scan of the brain to exclude raised intracranial pressure.

Spinal tumours

Spinal MRI

This is preferred to myelography as it is non-invasive, gives better results in terms of delineating local invasion in the transverse, sagittal, coronal and oblique views and defines the tumour's relation to surrounding anatomical structures.

Myelogram

This is mandatory for spinal primary tumours if MRI is not available.

Open biopsy

This will usually require a laminectomy and is especially difficult for anterior tumours, particularly of the thoracic spine when thoracotomy may be necessary.

Management

The skill and advice of a neurosurgeon should always be sought when planning investigation and treatment of such patients.

Surgery

This is the treatment of choice for all brain and spinal tumours as most are relatively radioresistant making them incurable by radiotherapy alone. Complete excision should be the goal of the neurosurgeon both to clear the tumour and to obtain adequate tissue for diagnosis. However, CNS tissue is not tolerant of trauma, is critical to normal body functioning and has no powers of regeneration, and so frequently the best that can be expected is surgical debulking. Tumours of the brain stem and pineal region are notoriously difficult to resect and are associated with high operative morbidity and mortality.

Radiotherapy

The CNS is not tolerant of high doses of radiation and therefore curative doses carry the risk of permanent neurological impairment. Radiotherapy has a complementary role to surgery, being ideal for eradicating small volume disease left behind after attempted surgical clearance, but may also be used to treat radiosensitive tumours arising in critical areas of the brain with a high expectation of cure, e.g. a dysgerminoma arising in the pineal region.

Chemotherapy

The blood–brain barrier may act as an obstacle to the free passage of chemotherapy drugs. Lipid soluble drugs such as the nitrosoureas BCNU and CCNU and very high doses of methotrexate do enter the brain in high concentrations, but only the very rare teratoma and dysgerminoma are potentially curable by chemotherapy and there is no useful role for chemotherapy in the other tumours. Intrathecal methotrexate and ara-C are of value in spinal deposits from lymphoma and leukaemia.

Supportive therapy

Dexamethasone 4–16 mg daily is very effective at relieving raised intra-cranial pressure. Prolonged usage does, however, lead to Cushingnoid symptoms and signs, oral candidiasis and proximal myopathy which may exacerbate neurological deficits. Mannitol intravenously is useful as an adjunct in an acute emergency.

Anticonvulsants should only be given for documented fits and patients with epilepsy or recent craniotomy should be advised not to drive until fit free during the daytime for 2 years or more. Many patients will have problems with the activities of everyday living due to neurological deficit and referral to a physiotherapist and occupational therapist is very important.

Astrocytoma

These arise from astrocytes in the brain or spinal cord, and are most common in adults but may arise during childhood. They are divided histologically into low grade (grades 1 and 2) and high grade (grades 3 and 4) which correlate with prognosis. Grade 4 tumours are termed glioblastoma multiforme. These comprise 50 per cent of astrocytomas, arising in adults with a peak incidence of 50 years. They are usually found in cerebral hemispheres, especially the frontal and temporal lobes, are extensively necrotic and haemorrhagic and have much associated oedema (Fig. 12.1). Tumours close to the midline may spread to the contralateral hemisphere via the corpus callosum or basal ganglia.

Management and prognosis

Surgery should be performed with the aim of complete macroscopic and microscopic resection. Post-operative radiotherapy will not be necessary for grade 1 tumours that have been completely resected. All other grades and incompletely resected grade 1 tumours should receive post-operative radiotherapy to maximize local control. Five year survival for grade 1 tumours is about 60 per cent, but high grade tumours have an extremely poor prognosis, with a median survival untreated of 3 months, 8 months when treated with radiotherapy, and a 1 year survival of 30 per cent. Apart from tumour grade, poor prognostic factors include advanced age, poor neurological performance status, limited surgical resection and no history of epilepsy.

Fig. 12.1 Contrast enhanced CT scan of a high grade glioma. Note the irregular area of oedema surrounding it and the invasion across the midline (courtesy of Dr R. Thomas).

Oligodendroglioma

These comprise only 5 per cent of gliomas, arising exclusively in adults with a mean age of 40 years. They are usually found in the cerebral hemispheres, particularly in the frontal lobes (50 per cent) and adjacent to the ventricles, and 20 per cent are bilateral. They are slow growing, well-circumscribed tumours, 40 per cent with foci of calcification, and unlike gliomas there is little associated oedema for their size. Patients often have a history of epilepsy or gradual deterioration in higher mental functions. Low grade tumours are compatible with a long survival after surgery alone which may be curative.

Meningioma

These comprise 15 per cent of intracranial tumours, are most common in adults and are the only CNS tumours which are more common in females. They arise from the arachnoid mater, adjacent to the major venous sinuses, the most common sites being the parasagittal region, olfactory groove, sphenoidal ridge and suprasellar region and may arise as an intradural extramedullary spinal tumour. They are benign, slow growing, well circumscribed, may erode overlying skull and 20 per cent are partly calcified. Primary treatment is surgery, with radiotherapy after incomplete excision and also for inoperable cases or recurrence after surgery. The prognosis is very good.

Pituitary tumours

Adenoma

Pituitary adenomas may be classified according to the staining characteristics of the cell of origin:

1. Chromophobe adenoma (50 per cent) – often large, forming the bulk of non-secretory tumours but may secrete prolactin.
2. Eosinophil adenoma (40 per cent) – much smaller than chromophobe adenomas and may secrete growth hormone or prolactin.
3. Basophil adenoma (10 per cent) – usually small, and may secrete ACTH, rarely TSH, LH or FSH.

Adenomas may present with headache or with more specific abnormalities.

The optic chiasm is a close anatomical relation of the pituitary fossa below and therefore suprasellar extension may lead to chiasmal compression and visual disturbance. Testing of the visual fields to confrontation and perimetry typically reveals a bitemporal hemianopia, although occasionally lateral extension may involve the cavernous sinuses resulting in a palsy of the 3rd, 4th and 6th cranial nerves. Examination of the fundi may reveal a pale disc consistent with optic atrophy.

Hypopituitism may occur as a result of compression of the pituitary gland adjacent to the tumour or pressure on the hypothalamus leading to a loss of hypothalamic regulation. Growth hormone secretion is the first to be impaired followed by the gonadotrophins. Diabetes insipidus indicates superior extension into the supra-optic nuclei.

Apart from pituitary hypofunction, prolactin may be elevated due to loss of the inhibitory hormone produced by the hypothalamus, and there may be disturbances in homeostasis such as loss of temperature regulation, disturbance of appetite and sleep.

The tumour cells may secrete excess amounts of hormones – eosinophilic adenomata may produce growth hormone or prolactin, chromophobes, prolactin and basophilic tumours ACTH.

Investigations

Referral to an endocrinologist

An expert endocrine assessment is mandatory before surgery and after treatment the patient will require lifelong follow-up and hormone replacement therapy.

Visual field perimetry

This is the most objective means of documenting visual field defects, and gives a hard copy which can be stored in the patient's notes for comparison at a later date.

AP/lateral SXR

This will document any bony expansion of the pituitary fossa (Fig. 12.2).

Fig. 12.2 Lateral skull X-ray showing marked erosion of the pituitary fossa by a large adenoma.

Fig. 12.3   CT scan showing a large tumour within the pituitary fossa.

CT or MRI of the pituitary fossa

These provide a detailed assessment of the pituitary fossa and local tumour spread, and are an indispensable part of planning surgery and radiotherapy (Fig. 12.3).

Treatment

Surgery

Hypophysectomy provides a tissue diagnosis and instant debulking, the aim being complete resection of the tumour. A transphenoidal approach is used but if there is much suprasellar or lateral extension a frontal approach will give greater access.

Radiotherapy

There is a high recurrence rate after surgery alone, but the addition of radiotherapy increases 10 year disease-free survival from 10 per cent to over 80 per cent.

Bromocriptine

This is a dopamine agonist which mimics the prolactin inhibitory hormone produced by the hypothalamus, and is of value in the treatment of prolactinoma when it may induce dramatic tumour regression.

Craniopharyngioma

This is very rare, usually arising in children, comprising 10 per cent of all childhood intracranial tumours. It is most common in Japan but rare in the US and Western Europe. It is a suprasellar tumour arising from nests of epidermoid cells in the pars tuberalis (Rathke's pouch), slow growing, benign, three-quarters being partly cystic and calcified. Presentation is as for pituitary adenomas and surgery is the treatment of choice with radiotherapy having the same role as for pituitary tumours. Prognosis is very good with an 80 per cent 5 year survival and 70 per cent 5 year disease-free survival.

Pineal tumours

Pinealoma

This is very rare, but is the most common pineal tumour with a peak incidence of 15–25 years. It is slow growing, well circumscribed and non-invasive and treated by surgical excision.

Pineoblastoma

This is even rarer and much more aggressive than pinealoma, CSF dissemination being a frequent complication.

Germ cell tumours

Teratomas and dysgerminomas (analogous to seminoma) may arise from islands of ectopic germ cells in the suprasellar region or pineal. The tumours are radiosensitive and chemosensitive but the prognosis is not as good as for their testicular counterparts. Serum and CSF α-foetoprotein and β human chorionic gonadotrophin measurements are useful to confirm diagnosis and monitor response to treatment.

Ependymoma

These comprise 10 per cent of childhood intracranial tumours with a peak incidence during the first decade of life. They arise throughout the CNS from cells lining ventricles, central canal of the spinal cord and choroid plexus, although the vast majority arise near the 4th ventricle, 40 per cent being supratentorial and 60 per cent infratentorial. They are well circumscribed, usually well differentiated, slow growing and may be calcified. Spread via CSF is well recognized, particularly if high grade and infratentorial. Combined surgery and radiotherapy give the greatest chance of local control, selected patients at high risk of CSF dissemination receiving radiotherapy to the craniospinal axis. The prognosis is a 5 year survival of about 50 per cent falling to 40 per cent at 10 years.

Medulloblastoma

This is the most common intracranial tumour in children (see Chapter 18), accounting for 20 per cent of intracranial tumours in the under 16s with 80 per cent arising in those under 15 years of age, most during the first decade. The cells of origin are foetal elements of the external granular layer of the cerebellum, and it is found centrally in the vermis in children, more laterally in hemispheres in young adults. There is a high risk of spread via CSF and it occasionally metastasizes outside CNS, usually to bone. It presents with cerebellar ataxia and/or obstructive hydrocephalus. Patients require a posterior fossa craniotomy and tumourectomy, a shunt being inserted to relieve raised intracranial pressure. Radiotherapy to the craniospinal axis is invariably indicated and the 5 year survival is approximately 50 per cent.

Chordoma

This very rare tumour presents in adult life, arising from notochord remnants in the axial skeleton anywhere from the sella turcica to the sacrum. In adults, these remnants persist in the nucleus pulposus of the intervertebral disc. Fifty per cent are sacrococcygeal, 35 per cent arise in the spheno-occipital region and 15 per cent in the vertebral column. They are slow growing, well circumscribed, gelatinous tumours with areas of haemorrhage and necrosis, often reaching a large size and causing compressive symptoms. They are locally invasive and may be confused with metastatic adenocarcinoma or chondrosarcoma, with less than 10 per cent metastasizing to distant sites. Radical excision should be attempted although it is rarely possible, and post-operative radiotherapy is necessary in the majority, giving a 50 per cent 5 year survival falling to 20 per cent at 10 years.

Haemangioblastoma

These are more common in children and form part of the von Hippel–Lindau syndrome. These are usually cerebellar in origin with the hemispheres affected more than the vermis. The tumour is slow growing, well circumscribed, and associated with polycythaemia due to ectopic secretion of erythropoietin.

Lymphoma (see chapters 16 and 20):

Primary cerebral lymphoma is very rare, and extracerebral involvement raises the possibility of secondary involvement of the brain. It is associated with AIDS but also occurs sporadically. It has a very poor prognosis, even in non-AIDS patients, with a median survival untreated of 3–4 months rising to 15 months after cranial radiotherapy. There is a tendency for CSF spread leading to involvement of the spinal cord and dura. In these circumstances, craniospinal irradiation may be of benefit. As with high grade gliomas, long term survivors are exceptional.

Metastases

These usually originate from lung, breast, kidney, colon, pancreas and melanoma. Lung cancer is the most common primary (50 per cent) where one-quarter of patients will have cerebral metastases at autopsy. They are usually multiple and most frequent in frontal and parietal lobes. They are usually well circumscribed and enhance on CT with intravenous contrast (Fig. 12.4). Craniotomy and biopsy may be considered if there is no known primary and no other malignant tissue to biopsy, or in a patient with previous cancer after a prolonged disease-free period. Potentially curable tumours such as germ cell tumours and lymphoma are managed aggressively. For carcinomas the treatment of choice is palliative radiotherapy which can safely be given in several fractions to limit hospital visits. Temporary epilation is inevitable. The median duration of improvement in such cases is 2–3 months, although some breast cancer patients survive for several years after diagnosis of cerebral metastases.

Fig. 12.4 CT brain scan showing a solitary metastasis. Note how well circumscribed it is compared to Figure 12.1 and the surrounding oedema.

13

Head and neck cancer

There are 2000 new cases of head and neck cancer and 900 deaths registered in the UK per annum. Nearly 90 per cent arise in the over 50s, the incidence increasing with age, and there is a strong male predominance. Incidence rates are greater in the north of England compared with the south, and the incidence and mortality rates are increasing. Worldwide, the highest incidence is in India and Sri Lanka where in some areas they are the most common cancers, comprising up to 40 per cent. Other pockets of high incidence include South America and the Bas-Rhin region of France (oral cancer), and Newfoundland (lip).

The head and neck contain the origins of the respiratory and gastrointestinal tracts, both of which are exposed to environmental carcinogens through the air we breathe and the food and drink we ingest. Each site will be dealt with individually, although cancer of the oral cavity will be described in detail as many of the basic principles are applicable to head and neck cancer in general.

Carcinoma of the oral cavity

This includes carcinoma of the lip, tongue, floor of mouth, buccal mucosa, hard palate, retromolar trigone and lower alveolus.

Aetiology

Inhalation of tobacco smoke from cigarettes, pipes and cigars is a major cause. As with lung cancer, the greater the amount smoked and the higher the tar content, the higher the risk. Chewing tobacco and 'snuff-dipping' carry a particularly high risk of carcinoma of the floor of the mouth where saliva pools.

Heavy alcohol consumption is a major risk factor and high alcohol mouthwashes have also been implicated. It acts synergistically with tobacco. Alcoholics also tend to have poor nutrition, and their low intake of vitamins A and C may add to their risk of developing cancer.

Carcinoma of the lip is more common in those with outdoor occupations where ultraviolet exposure is greater, and this accounts for the predominance of this tumour on the lower lip.

Physical trauma from poor dentition can lead to malignant transformation at the site of trauma, usually the lateral border of the tongue. Chronic heat trauma from claypipe smoking can lead to carcinoma of the lip.

Asians frequently chew betel nut to relieve indigestion and as a social habit, but this substance also contains carcinogens. This habit is easily detected by the dark brown staining between the teeth.

During the 19th century, chronic syphilitic glossitis was a major cause of carcinoma of the tongue. This has declined with the advent of effective antibiotic treatment of syphilis at an early stage and it is no longer justified to check routinely the syphilis serology in all patients with oral cavity cancer.

Pathology

The tumours may be frankly ulcerated, with raised, everted, nodular edges. They may also be papilliform or appear as subtle areas of superficial denudation of the mucosa. Synchronous primaries sometimes occur either in the oral cavity or elsewhere in the aerodigestive tract. The tumour may be secondarily infected, and there may be surrounding white plaques – leukoplakia – which are pre-malignant.

Ninety per cent are squamous carcinomas, the remainder being adenocarcinomas, mucoepidermoid carcinomas, adenoidcystic carcinomas, lymphomas and melanomas. *In situ* carcinoma and/or dysplasia may be seen in the surrounding mucosa.

Natural history

The tumours spread to adjacent subsites of the oral cavity and invade the deeper layers of the mucosa, reaching muscle in the case of the tongue and cheek, and even the underlying bone of the maxilla or mandible. Tumours of the lower alveolus tend to spread along the alveolus by insidious submucosal spread, so that their microscopic extent can be much greater than appreciated macroscopically.

A high proportion of patients have spread to the regional lymph nodes even when they are not palpable, e.g. 70 per cent in carcinoma of the tongue, the incidence being greater with increasing tumour size and increasingly undifferentiated tumours.

Haematogenous spread is uncommon at diagnosis and usually seen in the terminal phase of the disease, the lungs being the most common site followed by bone.

Symptoms

Many patients are asymptomatic, the tumour having been noticed at a routine dental examination, but some complain of soreness at the site of the tumour due to chronic superficial ulceration and occasionally the presentation is due to cervical lymph node enlargement. In locally advanced cases, pain may be more marked and may radiate to the ear, while a fungating tumour will lead to halitosis. Bulky tumours of the tongue

(Fig. 13.1) will interfere with mastication, swallowing and lead to slurred speech.

Signs

Patients frequently have physical signs consistent with heavy smoking and alcohol intake. Oral hygiene is often poor with an increased incidence of dental decay and gum disease, and this should be noted as it is relevant to the planning of radiotherapy. A thorough ENT examination is mandatory, preferably by an ENT surgeon. The primary tumour should be described in detail with respect to its position (preferably supplemented by a drawing), size and depth of invasion. Areas of leukoplakia should be sought and care taken to exclude another primary tumour. The tumour should be palpated with a gloved finger to complement inspection, feeling for induration and mucosal irregularity. All patients should have an indirect laryngoscopy. The neck should be palpated very carefully to detect enlarged lymph nodes, recording their distribution (preferably with a diagram), size, number, consistency, degree of tenderness and fixation to surrounding structures. It is frequent for small tender lymph nodes to be due to associated infection in the region of the tumour rather than lymph node metastases.

Differential diagnosis

Other causes of oral ulceration should be considered including:

1. Simple apthous ulceration.
2. Lichen planus.
3. Herpes simplex.
4. Syphilis.

Fig. 13.1 A large carcinoma of the tongue. Such tumours can interfere with speech and swallowing.

Investigations

Biopsy

A biopsy is essential to obtain tissue for histological analysis, and can be performed as an outpatient, by an ENT/oral surgeon.

Examination under general anaesthetic

This permits detailed palpation of the tumour to define its precise size, position and extent of local invasion.

Oral pantogram (OPG)

This is of value in excluding invasion of the mandible or maxilla, and provides a detailed survey of the teeth which will help plan any dental procedures that may be necessary prior to radiotherapy.

Fine needle aspirate of any enlarged lymph nodes

This should be performed in the outpatient clinic and the specimen sent for immediate cytology. As the result may make a substantial difference to the proposed treatment, it is worth repeating the aspiration if a negative lymph node is still clinically suspicious.

Chest X-ray

This should be performed in all cases to exclude obvious lung metastases, although suspicious areas should be reassessed by a CT scan of the chest.

Staging

The TNM staging is used:

Tis – Carcinoma *in situ*.
T0   – No evidence of primary.
Tx   – Primary cannot be assessed.
T1   – 2 cm or less in greatest dimension.
T2   – > 2 but not > 4 cm in greatest dimension.
T3   – > 4 cm in greatest dimension.
T4   – Invasion of deep (extrinsic) muscle of tongue, skin, cortical bone or maxillary sinus.
N0   – No regional lymphadenopathy.
N1   – Single ipsilateral node 3 cm or less in greatest dimension.
N2   – Single ipsilateral node > 3 but not > 6 cm in greatest dimension or multiple ipsilateral nodes not > 6 cm or bilateral/contralateral nodes not > 6 cm in greatest dimension.
N2a – Single ipsilateral node > 3 but not > 6 cm in greatest dimension.
N2b – Multiple ipsilateral nodes none > 6 cm in greatest dimension.
N2c – Bilateral/contralateral node(s) none > 6 cm in greatest dimension.
N3   – Any node > 6 cm in greatest dimension.

M0 – No distant metastases.
M1 – Distant metastases.

Treatment

Patients should ideally be seen at a joint clinic attended by a clinical oncologist and a head and neck surgeon. Patients should be advised to stop smoking and drinking alcohol to lessen the risk of mucositis during radiotherapy or chest infections after an anaesthetic.

Advice can be sought from:

1. A dietitian. Patients are frequently malnourished at presentation due to neglect, oral soreness or dysphagia and are therefore unlikely to tolerate either radical radiotherapy or surgery well. The patient may require a softer consistency of diet or liquid supplements. A liquidizer can be very useful.
2. A dentist. Patients having radiotherapy should have mild degrees of dental decay immediately dealt with by conservative measures, e.g. filling, while any teeth with serious decay will need extraction.

Radical

Surgery

The aim of surgery is to remove the primary tumour with a margin adequate to encompass all microscopic spread, and if necessary include an excision of the regional lymph nodes and reconstruct any major tissue deficits.

Surgery may be used as the sole primary treatment, combined with radiotherapy or as salvage for local recurrence following radical radiotherapy. Surgery may be the treatment of choice for locally advanced tumours, i.e. T3 and T4 tumours, as these are bulky tumours which may invade adjacent bone, making them difficult to eradicate by radiotherapy alone due to a high fraction of radioresistant hypoxic cells. There is also an increased risk of osteonecrosis after radiotherapy when the bone is invaded and this is a particularly difficult management problem. However, radical surgery may involve a major resection of tissue leading to severe functional morbidity. For example, resection of part of the tongue will result in some degree of dysarthria and possibly difficulty in mastication of food and swallowing, and such symptoms may severely compromise the patient's quality of life. Therefore T1, T2 and small bulk T3 tumours are usually best treated by radiotherapy with surgery reserved for local recurrence.

The surgeon may also elect to perform a radical dissection of the cervical lymph nodes when these are involved. This is a major procedure involving removal of the ipsilateral nodes en bloc together with the internal jugular vein (IJV) and some other tissues such as the sternocleidomastoid and accessory nerve. The IJV cannot be sacrificed bilaterally although a modified radical dissection may be performed on the contralateral side if necessary (IJV preserved). It may be a curative procedure and provides valuable staging and prognostic information. Radiotherapy is advised after neck dissection if three or more nodes are involved or if there is any evidence of extracapsular spread outside a lymph node.

Speech therapy is of value after major resections in the oral cavity, particularly of the tongue, floor of mouth and lips which may result in speech and swallowing difficulties.

Improvements in plastic surgical techniques have resulted in more patients being able to benefit from reconstructive procedures after radical cancer surgery. This has lessened considerably the functional morbidity experienced after major resections of the tongue and other structures of the oral cavity.

Radiotherapy

As with surgery, radiotherapy may be used as the sole primary treatment, combined with surgery or for salvage of local relapse after surgery, and can be used to treat all stages of local disease. It has the advantage of preserving the voice, speech, swallowing and tissues that surgery would sacrifice, and is therefore the treatment of choice for T1 and T2 tumours. Brachytherapy using radioactive needles (e.g. caesium), wire (e.g. iridium) or grains (e.g. gold) is superior to external beam radiotherapy in terms of local control and cosmetic outcome, but again is only suitable for early stage disease and inappropriate when there is a significant risk of lymph node involvement as it only treats the primary tumour. With external beam radiotherapy it is customary to include the first station lymph nodes adjacent to the primary tumour as a prophylactic measure to eradicate subclinical tumour deposits, whereas the whole cervical lymph node chain at risk is treated if there are palpable lymph node metastases. Radiotherapy gives poor local control when used alone for bulky T3 and T4 tumours.

Chemotherapy

The most active agents are methotrexate, 5FU and cisplatinum which in combination will give an objective response rate of 60–80 per cent. However, chemotherapy alone cannot be used with expectation of cure for metastatic disease, and adjuvant chemotherapy has no proven survival benefit.

Palliative

Surgery

Major resection is not justified for the palliation of symptoms in incurable cases due to the trauma sustained and the possibility of major post-operative morbidity with loss of function, but debulking may be necessary to avert respiratory obstruction or dysphagia. Tracheostomy may be indicated if there is upper airways obstruction as this is a particularly distressing symptom.

Radiotherapy

Radiotherapy may be used in cases of locally advanced disease even when the prospect of cure is low, being of value in relieving obstructive symptoms.

Tumour-related complications

Locally advanced tumours are often necrotic and infected which can lead to embarrassing halitosis, an unpleasant taste and local discomfort. A course of the appropriate antibiotic (usually metronidazole) and chlorhexidine mouthwash can help. Obstruction of the aerodigestive tracts is very distressing and warrants urgent consideration for a tracheostomy. Trismus, dysphonia, dysphagia and salivary fistulae are all recognized.

Treatment-related complications

Surgery

Difficulty in mastication, swallowing, dysarthria and dysphonia result from surgical resection of structures involved in these processes.

Poor healing is a particular problem following extensive surgery when the vascularity of the tissue has been compromised, especially if the tissues have been previously irradiated.

Osteomyelitis may complicate surgery when there has been a resection of bone (e.g. mandibulectomy) which has become secondarily infected. Treatment is with high doses of the appropriate antibiotic and further surgery may be required to remove the sequestrum.

Radiotherapy

The oral mucosa is very sensitive to radiation, the reaction beginning during the second week of radiotherapy as erythema and soreness, progressing to severe discomfort manifested as a fibrinous mucositis leading to dysphagia and difficulty in mastication. This can be lessened by advising patients to use a very soft tooth brush to avoid gingival trauma, regular mouthwashes to prevent secondary infection, avoiding smoking, alcohol, spicy foods, and food or drink that is very hot or very cold. Soluble aspirin 600 mg gargled and swallowed qds can relieve oral and oropharyngeal discomfort, while mucaine 10 ml qds sipped slowly can also help the latter. Local anaesthetic lozenges are also useful.

A dry mouth is very common during radiotherapy and may recover only partially or not at all. It results from radiation damage to the parotid salivary gland(s) at the site of radiation beam entry and/or exit from the oral cavity, predisposing the patient to dental caries, making swallowing difficult and exacerbating any radiation mucositis. Artificial saliva sprays are the treatment of choice but oral hygiene is also important.

Trismus is a late complication of both surgery and radiotherapy and is due to fibrosis in and around the temporomandibular joint leading to restriction of jaw opening and closing.

Osteonecrosis is a late complication of radiotherapy, usually affecting the mandible as the maxilla has a better blood supply. It may be precipitated by a dental infection or extraction many years after radiotherapy.

Prognosis

The prognosis varies greatly with site of origin, TNM stage and histological grade, and the reader should refer to a more specialized text for more detailed data. In general there is a high expectation of cure for all T1 and T2 tumours with a 5 year survival of 60–90 per cent, falling to less than 30 per cent for T4 tumours.

Screening/prevention

Dentists play a vital part in screening as they have the opportunity to inspect the oral cavity in many people on a regular basis, but unfortunately the people most at risk of cancer tend to be those who are least likely to attend a dentist. Long-term survivors should be kept under close surveillance in the clinic as many will develop second primaries, usually in the head and neck but also in the lung and gastrointestinal tract. Many cases of oral cavity cancer could be prevented by better patient education, i.e. by reducing smoking, and chewing tobacco and betel nut.

Rare tumours
Other rare carcinomas

The palate and oral mucosa contain a number of minor salivary glands which may result in mucoepidermoid carcinomas, adenocarcinomas and adenoidcystic carcinomas, which are treated by surgery with radiotherapy after incomplete excision or for inoperable tumours.

Kaposi's sarcoma

The oral cavity, particularly the palate, is a common site for this disease and should prompt serological testing to exclude AIDS (see Chapter 20).

Soft tissue and bone sarcomas

These are exceptionally rare but include leiomyosarcoma, rhabdomyosarcoma, fibrosarcoma, malignant fibrous histiocytoma, osteosarcoma and Ewing's sarcoma.

Metastases

Tumour cells may spread via the blood to the gingiva or lower alveolus, from which they may erode the overlying mucosa and mimic a primary carcinoma of the oral cavity. The lung is a common source of such metastases.

Future prospects

New techniques of radiotherapy scheduling (e.g. hyperfractionation, accelerated fractionation) are being evaluated with the expectation of improved local tumour control. There is no convincing benefit for neutrons or radiosensitizers in the treatment of these tumours.

Carcinoma of the oropharynx

The oropharynx comprises the tonsils, posterior third of the tongue, soft palate and posterior wall of the oropharynx. As the oropharynx is a direct extension of the oral cavity, tumours arising in this region are similar in their epidemiology, presentation and pathology. The structures do have a bilateral pattern of lymphatic drainage to the neck which should be considered when planning treatment. Radiotherapy is the preferred treatment for all but the earliest tumours as radical resection of the tonsil and adjacent tissues will compromise swallowing. It should be noted that the oropharynx is a site where lymphoid tissue is concentrated and where lymphoma may arise.

Carcinoma of the larynx

These tumours are more common in men, predisposed to by smoking, and 95 per cent are squamous carcinomas. All patients complaining of a hoarse voice which has persisted longer than a month should undergo indirect laryngoscopy to visualize directly the vocal cords. Glottic tumours arise on the vocal cords and present at an early stage as distortion of the vocal cords is rapidly manifest as dysphonia. Tumours may arise above the cords (supraglottic) or below the cords (subglottic). These tumours present later in their natural history as they grow insidiously and have to reach a large size before presenting with dysphagia, stridor or symptoms from direct invasion of the glottis. A tumour in the supraglottic larynx may lead to referred pain in the ipsilateral ear. The vocal cords have a poor lymphatic drainage and therefore lymph node metastases are less common at this site compared with a 70 per cent incidence from supraglottic tumours. Laryngeal tumours may be treated by surgery or radiotherapy. A partial or total laryngectomy will have the disadvantage of changing the quality of the voice, and therefore radiotherapy is preferred for T1, T2 and small bulk T3 tumours.

Carcinoma of the hypopharynx

The hypopharynx extends from the level of the tip of the epiglottis to the lower border of the cricoid and comprises the pyriform fossae, posterior pharyngeal wall and postcricoid region. The tumours are squamous carcinomas which tend to present late with dysphagia. There is an association with iron deficiency (Plummer–Vinson syndrome). The results of both radiotherapy and surgery alone are very poor, but the former is preferred unless the patient is physically fit for combined modality treatment.

Carcinoma of the nasopharynx

This disease has a marked geographical variation, being more common in the Far East, particularly Southern China where it is endemic. There is very strong evidence that in areas of high incidence the disease is related to infection with the Epstein–Barr virus (EBV). In endemic areas it has a peak incidence at a younger age (15–25 years v. 40–60 years in the UK) and a predominance of anaplastic tumours (squamous in the UK). Routes of spread include:

1. Nose – leads to epistaxis, nasal discharge and blockage.
2. Orbit – leads to diplopia.
3. Eustacian tube – blockage leads to deafness.
4. Cavernous sinus – causes palsies of cranial nerves 3, 4, 5 and 6.
5. Cribriform plate – leads to loss of smell.
6. Pterygoid muscles and parapharyngeal space – leads to inability to open jaw fully (trismus).

Seventy per cent will have overt or occult lymph node metastases with a tendency to bilateral involvement. The treatment of choice is radiotherapy. The prognosis for squamous carcinoma is poor with a 5 year survival of less than 20 per cent versus up to 50 per cent for other histological types.

Carcinoma of the paranasal sinuses

These are rare, sites of origin including the frontal, ethmoid, maxillary and sphenoid sinuses. They are usually squamous carcinomas, frequently presenting late as the symptoms are mistaken for those of chronic sinusitis. All too often, by the time of diagnosis they have spread beyond the bony walls of the sinus and have led to other symptoms due to local invasion of adjacent structures (Fig. 13.2) such as diplopia from orbital involvement, or epistaxis from nasal cavity involvement. They may also invade the cranial cavity. Radical surgery is hazardous due to adjacent vital organs and therefore radiotherapy is the treatment of choice. Approximately 40 per cent will survive 5 years after treatment.

(a)   (b)

Fig. 13.2   (a) A carcinoma of the maxillary antrum. Note the swelling of the cheek due to invasion outwards from the antrum anteriorly. There is also proptosis of the left eye indicating invasion of the orbit superior to the antrum (courtesy of Dr D. Tait). (b) CT scan of the head showing destruction of the facial bones by a large, soft tissue mass arising from the maxillary antrum.

Salivary gland tumours

The parotid gland forms the vast bulk of salivary gland tissue and therefore is the most common site for tumours, while the sublingual, submandibular and smaller glands distributed throughout the oral cavity are rarely involved. There are several variants.

Pleomorphic adenoma

This is the most common salivary gland tumour comprising 75 per cent, with a peak incidence of 30–50 years. It usually arises in the superficial lobe of the gland, is a benign tumour and therefore slow growing. There is never any associated facial nerve weakness – this feature should always suggest carcinoma or lymphoma. All cases are treated by superficial parotidectomy. Post-operative radiotherapy is indicated if there is capsular rupture at the time of surgery or incomplete microscopic clearance. There is a small risk of transformation of a recurrence into a carcinoma.

Adenolymphoma

This is a benign, slow growing tumour most commonly arising in the lower pole of the superficial lobe of the parotid, and is bilateral in 5 per cent. The treatment of choice is surgery.

Carcinoma

This usually arises *de novo* but may develop in a pleomorphic adenoma. It may be distinguished clinically from benign tumours when a facial nerve palsy is present. Variants include:

1. Adenoidcystic carcinoma – slow growing and has a tendency for invasion along nerves and into the cranial cavity.
2. Acinic cell carcinoma arising from serous cells.
3. Mucoepidermoid carcinoma arising from mucin cells.
4. Adenocarcinoma.
5. Squamous carcinoma - must be distinguished from a metastasis.
6. Undifferentiated carcinoma.

The treatment of choice is resection of the lobe of origin followed by radiotherapy to the parotid. Five year survival varies between 20 and 80 per cent depending on tumour type and histological grade.

Lymphoma

The parotid is a common site of extranodal non-Hodgkin's lymphoma. Localized disease can be treated by radiotherapy, with chemotherapy used for more advanced disease.

Orbital tumours

These are all very rare, presenting due to a mass effect leading to proptosis and diplopia. Benign tumours include hemangioma, leiomyoma, rhabdomyoma, lipoma, fibroma, meningioma, neurofibroma, schwannoma, pseudotumour and 'malignant' granuloma, e.g. Wegener's granulomatosis. Malignant tumours include gliomas, rhabdomyosarcoma, leiomyosarcoma, malignant fibrous histiocytoma, fibrosarcoma, osteosarcoma, chondrosarcoma, Ewing's sarcoma, lymphoma, histiocytosis X, melanoma, nephroblastoma and metastases.

Tumours within the eye itself are also very rare, presenting with visual loss and strabismus. Benign tumours include naevi, leiomyoma, haemangioma and hamartoma. Malignant tumours include retinoblastoma, medulloepithelioma, melanoma and metastases.

With both sites, optimum management will preserve vision in the affected eye as much as possible, and usually comprises radiotherapy alone, surgery alone or combined modality treatment.

14

Endocrine tumours

Thyroid cancer

Epidemiology

There are 800 new cases of thyroid cancer and 400 deaths registered in the UK per annum. The overall incidence increases with age, papillary, follicular and medullary types often arising in young adults while anaplastic cancers are usually seen in the elderly. There is a female predominance and a particularly high incidence in Iceland, Israel and Hawaii.

Aetiology

Ionizing radiation is a recognized aetiological agent. Radiation-induced cancers have a latency of 5–40 years, with a peak 15 years after exposure. Radiation induces papillary cancer, which has been described following childhood irradiation for thymic hyperplasia, ringworm, cervical lymphadenitis and in atomic bomb survivors.

A higher incidence of follicular cancer has been noted in endemic goitre areas where there is a dietary deficiency of iodine, while a higher incidence of papillary cancer is seen in areas where there is an excess of iodine in the diet.

Multiple endocrine adenomatosis (MEA) is a dominantly inherited condition, type 1 being occasionally associated with differentiated thyroid cancer while type 2 is associated with medullary cancer which is more often multifocal and presents at a younger age than its sporadic counterpart.

Rare associations include:

1. Dyshormonogenesis.
2. Pendred's syndrome (goitre and nerve deafness at birth).
3. Gardener's syndrome (polyposis of the bowel, osteomas and sebaceous cysts).
4. Cowden's disease (multiple haematomas).

Pathology

The tumour usually appears as a firm, well-circumscribed lump, often with a pseudocapsule of compressed thyroid tissue at its periphery. The cut surface will have a characteristic glistening appearance of colloid if there is a significant follicular element. There may be haemorrhage and necrosis in anaplastic tumours, and it may be multifocal. Follicular, papillary and medullary cancers may grow very slowly over many years, while anaplastic cancers are usually fast growing and locally invasive. Tumours may arise in ectopic thyroid tissue in the tongue, a thyroglossal cyst, sublingual, infrahyoid, pretracheal, mediastinal and pericardial regions.

Microscopically, thyroid cancer is characterized by invasion of the capsule and/or thyroid vasculature. There are four main types:

Papillary carcinoma (50 per cent)

The presence of papillae is diagnostic although there may be a strong follicular component.

Follicular carcinoma (20 per cent)

This must be distinguished from an adenoma. It is usually well differentiated with colloid held within follicles and there are no papillary elements.

Anaplastic carcinoma (25 per cent)

The tumour is very poorly differentiated, usually with no identifiable follicular elements.

Medullary carcinoma (4 per cent)

This arises from the parafollicular ('C') cells, with the inherited form often multifocal in origin. Amyloid may be identified within the stroma and immunocytochemistry will be positive for the hormone calcitonin.

Squamous carcinoma, clear cell carcinoma and Hurthle cell carcinoma are also recognized.

Natural history

The tumour initially spreads within the lobe of origin, contained by the capsule, but may then invade the contralateral lobe via the isthmus. Capsular invasion will lead to infiltration of surrounding structures such as the trachea, larynx, recurrent laryngeal nerves and skin.

Papillary and medullary carcinomas have a propensity to metastasize to lymph nodes, the affected groups comprising the deep cervical, supraclavicular and paratracheal chains.

All may give rise to distant metastases, the lung being the most common site, followed by the skeleton, liver, skin, brain and kidney. Lung metastases are often very numerous and small, sometimes giving a 'snowstorm' appearance. Follicular and anaplastic variants are the types most often associated with distant metastases.

Symptoms

The most common presentation is with a painless solitary lump in the neck. Some patients complain of a hoarse voice, which raises the suspicion of extracapsular extension leading to pressure on one or both of the recurrent laryngeal nerves innervating the vocal cords. Dysphagia may be noticed if the tumour is very large and causing extrinsic compression of the pharynx or upper oesophagus, and may suggest retrosternal extension if the neck mass is small. Patients with medullary carcinoma may complain of diarrhoea which is probably due to secretion of prostaglandins by the tumour.

Signs

The patient will be euthyroid. The thyroid lump is usually confined to one side of the neck moving with swallowing and protrusion of the tongue, non-tender, firm/hard in consistency and well circumscribed. Stridor may be heard due to either recurrent laryngeal nerve involvement or extrinsic tracheal compression. Vocal cord palsy may be confirmed by indirect laryngoscopy (IDL). Extracapsular invasion may lead to loss of the normal laryngeal mobility. Lymphadenopathy may be palpable in the deep cervical and supraclavicular regions, while anaplastic tumours may invade the overlying skin to produce induration, erythema and nodularity.

Differential diagnosis

This includes:

1. Benign tumours of thyroid, e.g. adenoma.
2. Other malignant tumours of thyroid, e.g. lymphoma, fibrosarcoma.
3. Metastases, e.g. carcinoma of the lung, hypernephroma, melanoma.

Investigations

Chest X-ray

This should be performed in all patients to exclude pulmonary metastases.

Thoracic inlet X-rays

These are useful for detecting any significant retrosternal extension of tumour.

Thyroid ultrasound and fine needle aspiration (FNA)

Carcinoma will give rise to a solid nodule rather than a cystic one and in either case FNA should be performed to obtain a cytological diagnosis.

FNA of enlarged lymph nodes

This is essential to distinguish reactive lymph node enlargement from metastatic infiltration.

Open thyroid biopsy

This is only required in inoperable tumours when a FNA has proven negative or given an equivocal histological diagnosis.

Isotope thyroid scan

In the case of thryoid cancer, administration of a tracer dose of Technecium[99] or Iodine[131] will give rise to a cold spot relative to the surrounding functioning thyroid tissue, giving useful information to the surgeon regarding its location and extent. Functioning adenomas will produce a hot spot.

CT scan of the neck

This is not routinely required, but may be of value in assisting the surgeon to make a decision regarding operability of a large mass or when retrosternal extension is suspected.

Serum calcitonin

This should be performed in any patient suspected of having medullary carcinoma, e.g. if there is a family history of thyroid carcinoma at a young age or associated diarrhoea. These patients should also be screened for other MEA type 2 tumours, i.e. parathyroid adenomas (serum calcium and phosphate), phaeochromocytoma (urinary vanillylmandelic acid).

Staging

TX   – Primary tumour cannot be assessed.
T0   – No evidence of tumour.
T1   – Unilateral tumour. Thyroid mobile.
T1s – Single nodule.
T1m – Multiple nodules.
T2   – Bilateral tumour. Thyroid mobile.
T2s – Single tumour of isthmus.
T3   – Extension beyond gland indicated by fixation of thyroid or infiltration of surrounding structures.

Treatment

All patients should have some form of thyroid ablation followed by physiological hormone replacement therapy to prevent hypothyroidism and maintain TSH at very low ('suppressed') levels to minimize the likelihood of recurrence of a TSH-dependent tumour.

Radical

Surgery

This may be curative when used alone, all patients requiring a total thyroidectomy with the aim of removing all thyroid tissue and any extracapsular extension, taking care to preserve the parathyroid glands and recurrent laryngeal nerves if possible. A radical neck dissection should be undertaken when there is overt lymphatic invasion.

Radiotherapy

Radioiodine is concentrated in the thyroid gland and can therefore be used for the diagnosis of locoregional and metastatic disease, for the ablation of a thyroid remnant and/or tumour persisting after surgery, and as a means of detecting early relapse. It is concentrated by normal thyroid tissue, 70–80 per cent of well-differentiated thyroid carcinomas and their metastases (Fig. 14.1). Radioiodine is given as an oral preparation using strict radiation protection procedures, with the large doses used for ablation of thyroid and tumour being given as an inpatient. It emits β particles (electrons) with a tissue range of only 2 mm, and it is these that ablate the thyroid/tumour. It also emits low energy γ photons which are a radiation hazard to staff and visitors but allow external monitoring of the distribution, concentration and excretion of the isotope.

Radioiodine is given primarily to destroy any remaining normal thyroid tissue. If scans demonstrate any distant metastases, further doses are given to concentrate higher radiation doses at those sites. Most patients will require one to three such treatments, six being the maximum possible.

External beam irradiation to the neck is used when there is residual papillary or follicular carcinoma in the neck that is not concentrating Iodine[131], and is necessary in all cases of anaplastic carcinoma and incompletely excised medullary carcinomas.

Palliative

Surgery

Tracheostomy is occasionally necessary, particularly with anaplastic tumours causing tracheal compression and when there are bilateral palsies of the recurrent laryngeal nerves leading to total vocal cord paralysis and upper respiratory obstruction.

Radiotherapy

Death from asphyxiation due to a rapidly growing anaplastic carcinoma is particularly unpleasant and distressing and under such circumstances, even if the patient has distant metastases, radiotherapy to the neck is justified.

Chemotherapy

Chemotherapy has no role in the curative treatment of thyroid cancer. Patients with anaplastic carcinoma and symptoms refractory to all other treatments may be considered for palliative chemotherapy. Adriamycin is the most active agent. Responses are short-lived and toxicity considerable.

Hormone therapy

Elderly patients unfit for surgery with small, well-differentiated tumours may be treated by thyroxine alone at a dose sufficient to suppress TSH, as

(a)

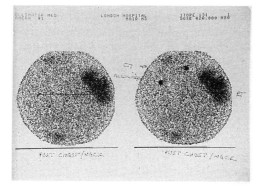

(b)

Fig. 14.1   (a) Chest X-ray showing a pleural metastasis in the left upper zone from a follicular carcinoma of the thyroid. (b) Iodine[131] uptake scan showing increased uptake (dark) in the corresponding region.

the natural history of the disease is likely to be greater than the patients' natural life expectancy.

Tumour-related complications

Respiratory obstruction is seen with anaplastic carcinomas due to extrinsic compression of the trachea or bilateral damage to the recurrent laryngeal nerves, while dysphagia may result from extrinsic compression of the cervical oesophagus and/or retrosternal extension. Superior vena caval obstruction is a rare complication associated with a large retrosternal tumour.

Treatment-related complications

Surgery

Specific complications include risk of secondary haemorrhage during the post-operative period, laryngeal oedema, hypoparathyroidism (hypocalcaemia leading to perioral paraesthesiae, tetany, Trousseau's sign, Chvostek's sign) and vocal cord palsy due to damage to the recurrent laryngeal nerves leading to dysphonia and respiratory obstruction.

Radiotherapy

External beam irradiation to the neck will result in an acute radiation laryngitis characterized by sore throat, dysphagia and dysphonia. Late complications include chronic laryngeal oedema, intense subcutaneous fibrosis leading to restricted neck movements and radiation chondritis of the tracheal cartilage rings.

Radioiodine

Severe adverse reactions to radioiodine are rare. Possible complications include nausea, acute parotitis, sore throat due to radiation laryngitis, acute pneumonitis if there are miliary lung metastases, myelosuppression, leukaemogenesis and induction of cancer elsewhere (there is some uptake in the salivary glands, stomach, colon and bladder).

Hormone replacement therapy

Inappropriate dosage or poor patient compliance may lead to either hypothyroidism or hyperthyroidism.

Prognosis

Differentiated thyroid cancer has a good prognosis. Papillary carcinoma has the best prognosis of all with a 10 year survival of more than 90 per cent, followed by follicular carcinoma (80 per cent) and medullary carcinoma (60–70 per cent). Most patients with anaplastic carcinoma will die within 6 months after diagnosis. Children have an extremely good prognosis, young adults fare better than the elderly and women fare better than men, again reflecting the incidence of differentiated thyroid cancer in these groups. Extra-capsular invasion, lymphatic invasion and distant metastases are poor prognostic signs.

Screening/prevention

Patients developing medullary carcinoma of the thyroid have a significant risk of having MEA2, particularly if aged 20–40 years with a multifocal carcinoma, and screening of their first degree relatives by measuring serum calcitonin may detect occult carcinomas which can be easily cured by surgery.

Rare tumours

Lymphoma

This comprises less than 2 per cent of extranodal lymphomas, with a median age at presentation of 65 years and a female predominance. It is invariably a non-Hodgkin's lymphoma, usually diffuse high grade and may be preceded by Hashimoto's thyroiditis. It is staged and treated using the same principles as for lymphoma elsewhere and has a 5 year survival of about 40 per cent.

Future prospects

It may be possible to conjugate thyroglobulin with radioactive isotopes to act as tracers or therapeutic agents for tumours that do not take up radioiodine.

Tumours of the parathyroid glands

These are rare and may be part of MEA1 or 2. Adenomas are usually impalpable, solitary and present with hyperparathyroidism (high serum calcium, low serum phosphate, hyperchloraemic metabolic acidosis, evidence of subperiosteal bone resorption on plain radiographs, e.g. of phalanges). The glands can be imaged by radioisotope imaging using a Technecium[99] scan (images the thyroid) followed by a Thallium[201] scan (images both the thyroid and the parathyroids), subtraction of the two images giving an image of the parathyroids alone. Ultrasound or MRI of the neck are alternatives, and venous sampling for parathyroid hormone is useful for tumours that cannot be visualized. Parathyroidectomy is the sole treatment. Carcinoma is extremely rare.

Tumours of the adrenal glands

Tumours of the adrenal gland are rare, accounting for approximately 100 deaths per annum.

Phaeochromocytoma

This is a very rare tumour arising from the autonomic cells of the adrenal medulla, with a peak incidence at 35–55 years but may occur from infancy to old age. Recognized associations include:

1. Multiple endocrine adenomatosis types 2a and 2b.
2. Neurofibromatosis (seen in 5 per cent presenting with sporadic or familial phaeocromocytomas. One per cent of patients presenting with neurofibromatosis have phaeochromocytomas).
3. Previous neuroblastoma.
4. Hippel-Von Lindau syndrome.

Ninety-nine per cent are found in the abdomen or pelvis, 90 per cent of these in the adrenal medulla, the most common extra-adrenal site being the organ of Zuckerkandl adjacent to the aortic bifurcation. Other sites include the sympathetic chain, bladder, thorax (usually paravertebral) and carotid arch. The tumours may be very small or weigh several kilograms, are well circumscribed, slow growing, with 10 per cent bilateral (70 per cent in familial cases), 90 per cent benign and 10 per cent malignant. They are rich in lipid and therefore yellow in cut section. Phaeochromocytomas arise from chromaffin cells of neural crest origin. The cells therefore stain with chrome salts, enzymes such as DOPA decarboxylase and contain neurosecretory granules. As most tumours are benign, local invasion is unusual although malignant tumours may infiltrate the underlying kidney and retroperitoneum. Lymphatic spread is unusual but malignant tumours may spread to lung, bone and liver. The classical presentation is with paroxysms of headache, postural dizziness, feelings of apprehension and fear, pallor, sweating, tremor, chest pain and palpations. Attacks last minutes to hours and are followed by a feeling of exhaustion and muscle pain, and may be precipitated by emotion, exertion, posture, bending, pressure on tumour, foods or handling of tumour at operation. Half the patients have sustained hypertension while 70 per cent have postural hypotension. Investigations include:

1. Urinary vanillylmandelic acid (VMA) and catecholamine estimations – these are estimated from a 24 hour urine collection, and are useful screening tests during investigation of malignant hypertension. Urinary VMA is elevated in phaeochromocytoma, while high levels of adrenaline suggest an adrenal origin, high levels of noradrenaline suggest an extra-adrenal tumour, and high levels of dopamine suggest a malignant phaeochromocytoma.
2. CT scan – this is the best investigation for delineating site and size of primary and excluding gross tumour in the contralateral adrenal, but is limited by its resolution of 0.5–1 cm which will miss some tumours.
3. Selective venous sampling – this localises radiologically occult tumours, identifying their venous drainage using multiple venous samples which are tested for catecholamines.
4. Selective arteriography – this is also of value when planning surgery as phaeochromocytomas have a rich vascular supply, but it may

precipitate a hypertensive crisis.

5. Metaiodobenzylguanidine (mIBG) imaging – this technique is not widely available, but is of benefit in staging patients with malignant tumours, the iodine moiety being radioactive Iodine[131] and therefore detectable by a gamma camera to give a whole body image.

Adrenalectomy is the treatment of choice, expert anaesthetic advice and pre-operative α and β blockade (e.g. phenoxybenzamine and propranolol) being necessary as the tumour will be handled leading to a release of catecholamines. At laparotomy it is important to inspect the contralateral adrenal for a second primary. In inoperable cases, phenoxybenzamine is a useful medical therapy, being an α adrenergic receptor blocker. Alpha methyl tyrosine inhibits hydroxylation of tyrosine to DOPA, an intermediate compound in the synthesis of catecholamines, and is a more toxic alternative. External beam radiotherapy and chemotherapy have no role in the curative treatment of these tumours, although the former is of value in palliating local symptoms from metastases and mIBG can be used to treat metastatic disease if the tumour concentrates enough of it. With regard to prognosis, 75 per cent will be cured by surgery alone, and even patients with malignant tumours may survive for many years, death often resulting from cardiovascular complications, e.g. myocardial infarction, cerebrovascular accident.

Adrenal cortex tumours

Benign tumours are common at autopsy in the general population, but may be part of MEA type 1 disease. Most are non-functioning, the majority of functioning tumours arising in females. Of functioning tumours, those arising in prepubertal patients are virilizing, while those in postpubertal patients tend to produce Cushing's syndrome although Conn's syndrome (primary hyperaldosteronism) may also result. A CT scan will delineate the primary tumour if greater than 1 cm in diameter, although angiography is more sensitive, and treatment is by adrenalectomy.

Malignant tumours are rare, with a slight female predominance, arising at a younger age than most other carcinomas (median 35–55 years). Half are functioning and as with benign tumours are more frequent in females. Presentation is with vague abdominal symptoms, and up to one-third have signs of endocrine dysfunction, usually a combination of Cushing's syndrome and virilism. Half have metastatic disease at presentation, haematogenous spread occurring to lung and liver. Investigation and treatment is as for benign tumours. In advanced disease metyrapone (250 mg–1 g qds) is useful for palliation of Cushing's syndrome by inhibiting 11 β hydroxylase but it may exacerbate virilism and physiological glucocorticoid replacement is necessary. Aminoglutethimide may be added if control is insufficient. An alternative is o'p'DDD which causes necrosis and atrophy of normal adrenal tissue and differentiated carcinoma cells, reducing steroid output in 70 per cent and giving objective tumour regression in one-third, although response is slow and glucocorticoid cover necessary.

Carcinoid tumours

Epidemiology

These are rare tumours arising at a younger age than carcinomas, with a peak incidence at about 50 years. There is no significant sex predominance or geographical pattern.

Aetiology

It may be a feature of multiple endocrine adenomatosis type 1.

Pathology

The primary tumour is often small compared with the bulk of liver metastases and symptoms of the carcinoid syndrome. They usually arise submucosally and appear as a nodule, often red/brown in colour, yellow in cut section, may be multifocal, and unlike carcinomas ulceration is uncommon. Carcinoid is most common in the small bowel – 90 per cent arise in the ileum, particularly the terminal segment, 7 per cent in the jejunum, 2 per cent in the duodenum and 2 per cent in a Meckel's diverticulum, but may arise elsewhere in the gastrointestinal tract, e.g. stomach, colon, rectum and other midline structures such as thyroid, lung, bladder, testes, ovaries, common bile duct and pancreas. An encasement reaction characterized by a massive fibrous stroma may occur when the tumour reaches the mesentery and this predisposes to bowel obstruction.

Carcinoids arise from APUD (amine precursor uptake and decarboxylation) cells which are derived from the neural crest. Midgut-derived carcinoids characteristically stain with and reduce silver salts (argentaffin reaction), others stain with silver but cannot reduce it (argyrophilic reaction, e.g. gastric and bronchial carcinoids), while hindgut-derived carcinoids do not take up silver. Immunocytochemistry indicates staining for cromogranin which is useful when the diagnosis is in doubt.

Natural history

The tumours frequently behave in a benign manner and local infiltration of surrounding tissues is unusual.

In contrast to a carcinoma, lymphatic spread is uncommon. Haematogenous spread is usually to the liver as most tumours will arise in the portal circulation. Ileal tumours frequently metastasize, especially if more than 2 cms in diameter, while appendiceal, rectal and bronchial carcinoids rarely metastasize. The metastases are characteristically multiple and bulky compared with the primary, and may undergo spontaneous necrosis. The skeleton is sometimes a site of distant metastases.

Symptoms

Symptoms depend on the site and size of the tumour. Carcinoids are often found incidentally at appendicectomy, when they are almost invariably benign and therefore very rarely metastasize to the liver. The patient may notice an abdominal mass if the tumour is large and superficial, or experience colicky abdominal pain if there is significant stenosis of the bowel lumen. Ultimately there may be symptoms of subacute small bowel obstruction. Bronchial carcinoids present with haemoptysis or bronchial obstruction leading to recurrent chest infections.

Carcinoid syndrome arises when there are liver metastases, so that the vasoactive tumour products, particularly 5-hydroxytryptamine (5HT, serotonin), reach the systemic circulation, or in tumours arising outside the portal circulation. It comprises:

1. Flushing – distribution may vary with site of primary.
2. Weals – due to release of histamine.
3. Lacrimation.
4. Facial oedema.
5. Tachycardia, hypotension.
6. Wheezing.
7. Diarrhoea, borborygmi, abdominal colic and weight loss.

A given patient with liver metastases will not necessarily have all these symptoms and may complain of hepatic pain if a large subcapsular metastasis infarcts. Attacks may be precipitated by alcohol, stress, emotion, ingestion of food, infusion of calcium, noradrenaline or pentagastrin.

Signs

The patient with advanced disease often looks remarkably well bearing in mind the bulk of liver metastases. The patient may appear malnourished if diarrhoea has been a particular problem, an abdominal mass may be palpable or there may be signs in the chest of pulmonary collapse/consolidation depending on the site of the primary tumour. Hepatomegaly is expected in patients with carcinoid syndrome. Auscultation of the heart may reveal tricuspid or pulmonary valve disease, although left-sided cardiac lesions have been described with bronchial carcinoids.

Differential diagnosis

Other tumours arising at the site of the carcinoid should be considered, although none produce a syndrome akin to carcinoid when there are liver metastases. It should be noted that carcinomas at other sites may produce a carcinoid syndrome due to 5HT production, e.g. medullary carcinoma of the thyroid, small cell lung cancer.

Investigations

Urinary 5-hydroxyindoleacetic acid (5HIAA)

Twenty-four hour urinary 5HIAA is elevated in those with carcinoid syndrome, reflecting metabolism of 5-hydroxytryptamine. A false positive result may be obtained if the diet at the time of urine collection is rich in bananas, pineapples, advocados or walnuts. Apart from 5HT, carcinoids may produce histamine, kallikrein, motilin, enteroglucagon, neurotensin, substance P, prostaglandins, insulin, ACTH, glucagon, parathyroid hormone and calcitonin, most of which can be assayed if clinically relevant.

CT scan of liver and site of primary

This defines the extent of primary and will exclude liver metastases.

Hepatic angiography

This is of value if resection of liver metastases is planned.

Staging

There is no formal staging system in routine clinical use.

Treatment

Radical

Surgery

The primary tumour should be completely excised as this offers the only chance of long-term cure. Radical lymph node resection is unnecessary, although obviously enlarged nodes should be cleared to ensure a complete resection of the tumour.

Palliative

Dietary advice

Referral to a dietitian may help the patient to avoid ingestion of substances which may precipitate an attack of flushing and permit modification of the diet to lessen diarrhoea and protein-losing enteropathy.

Surgery

In patients with symptoms from one large liver metastasis or multiple metastases confined to one lobe of the liver, resection may be justified to reduce tumour bulk, thereby reducing secretion of vasoactive peptides and therefore palliating symptoms.

Radiotherapy

Carcinoids are not sensitive to radiation, although low doses of radiation are useful for the palliation of skeletal metastases.

Pharmacological measures

Codeine phosphate (30–60 mg tds) or loperamide (up to 16 mg daily) are both useful for the treatment of diarrhoea. Other drugs used for the palliation of symptoms refractory to more conventional measures include:

1. Parachlorophenylalanine – blocks conversion of tryptophan to 5-hydroxytryptophan, a precursor of 5HT.
2. Cyproheptadine – blocks action of 5HT on its receptors.
3. Ketanserin – a $5HT_2$ receptor antagonist.
4. Somatostatin.

Hepatic arterial embolization

This may be of benefit in up to 80 per cent with symptomatic hepatic metastases, with palliation lasting up to 3 years. This procedure may be repeated as necessary.

Chemotherapy

Streptozotocin is the most active chemotherapy agent with a partial response rate of 30 per cent.

Tumour-related complications

As with any other gastrointestinal tumour perforation, obstruction or intussusseption may all occur. Ectopic hormone production is recognized, the tumour producing growth hormone releasing hormone leading to acromegaly or ACTH leading to Cushing's syndrome. Pellagra is a rare syndrome characterized by dermatitis in sun-exposed areas, diarrhoea and dementia, and is due to the tumour consuming tryptophan which is a precursor for nicotinic acid.

Treatment-related complications

All cytoreductive treatments can release large amounts of vasoactive substances and therefore patients with bulky tumours should be pretreated with parachlorophenylalanine and cyproheptadine to avoid a serotonergic crisis.

Prognosis

Carcinoid tumours are usually very slow growing so that even patients with heavy metastatic burdens may survive for many years. Appendiceal carcinoids have an excellent prognosis as they are small, easily removed and rarely metastasize.

Multiple endocrine adenomatosis (MEA)

Type 1

Described by Werner, it is dominantly inherited. Involved glands include:

1. Parathyroids (90 per cent) – hyperplasia or adenoma.
2. Pancreatic islets (80 per cent) – adenoma, carcinoma or more rarely diffuse hyperplasia.
3. Anterior pituitary (65 per cent) – adenomas.
4. Adrenal cortex (38 per cent) – hyperplasia or adenoma.

    Carcinoid is also a rare association.

Type 2

Originally described by Sipple, with an autosomal dominant inheritance. Involved glands include:

1. Parafollicular cells of thyroid – medullary carcinomas.
2. Adrenal medulla – phaeochromocytoma.
3. Parathyroids – hyperplasia or adenoma.

Subtype A has no mucocutaneous features while subtype B is characterized by multiple small subcutaneous or submucosal neuromas of the oral cavity and lips, autonomic ganglioneuromatosis, and Marfanoid habitus.

Mixed MEA

This demonstrates features of both types 1 and 2.

15

Sarcomas

Soft tissue sarcomas

Epidemiology

Soft tissue sarcomas are rare tumours with around 1000 cases reported in the UK each year divided equally between men and women. In children the predominant tumour is a juvenile rhabdomyosarcoma which will be considered in the section on paediatric tumours having very different characteristics to the soft tissue sarcomas of adults. In adults these tumours can occur at any age, the incidence being slightly more common in the 50 to 70 year age group.

Aetiology

Usually there is no identifiable cause but the following factors may be of importance:

Chronic mechanical irritation

Sarcomas can be induced in animal models but this does not appear important in humans.

Radiation

A small number of sarcomas are undoubtedly related to previous thera-peutic irradiation with tumours developing several years after exposure.

Familial

Forming part of the LiFraumeni syndrome where they are associated with tumours of breast, brain, adrenal cortex and leukaemias in close relatives under the age of 45 years.

Also seen in patients with Von Recklinghausen's syndrome of familial neurofibromatosis with malignant change within pre-existing neuro-fibromata occurring.

Chemical

Angiosarcoma is associated with vinyl chloride exposure.

Pathology

Sites for soft tissue sarcomas are shown in Table 15.1.

Macroscopically soft tissue sarcomas are often large fleshy tumour masses with associated haemorrhage and necrosis. They are seen to invade local soft tissues, nerves and blood vessels.

Microscopic classification of soft tissue sarcomas is based on the finding of recognizable connective tissue elements within the tumour. The basis of the diagnosis is the finding of malignant spindle cells which may form characteristic patterns as in a fibrosarcoma when a 'herringbone' pattern is described and malignant fibrous histiocytoma when a 'cartwheel' pattern may be seen. A classification of the soft tissue sarcomas is shown in Table 15.2

Histological grade is an important prognostic feature of sarcomas and a three point scale is used to describe the degree of differentiation. This

Table 15.1   Distribution by site for soft tissue sarcomas

Limbs	
upper	15%
lower	40%
Retroperitoneum	20%
Viscera (bladder, bowel, uterus)	10%
Trunk	10%
Head and neck	4%

Table 15.2   Classification of soft tissue sarcomas

Sarcoma subtype	Tissue type	Features
Malignant Fibrous Histiocytoma (MFH)	Histiocytic	Most common sarcoma, especially legs, buttocks and retroperitoneum
Fibrosarcoma	Fibrous tissue	Thigh most common
Liposarcoma	Fat	Lower extremity and retroperitoneum
Rhabdomyosarcoma	Skeletal muscle	Adult forms are alveolar or pleomorphic
Leiomyosarcoma	Smooth muscle	Uterus and gastrointestinal tract common, also limbs and retroperitoneum
Neurogenic sarcoma (Neurofibrosarcoma)	Neural tissue	Arise within large nerves, e.g. sciatic, median, spinal roots
Synovial sarcoma	Uncertain	Arise around joints, especially thigh, foot, knee
Angiosarcoma	Blood vesels	Scalp, breast, liver
Lymphangiosarcoma	Lymph vessels	Sites of chronic lymphoedema, postmastectomy arm

must, however, be interpreted in the light of the cell type. For example, angiosarcoma will usually appear well differentiated but is usually a highly malignant tumour. Similarly, virtually all synovial sarcomas can be regarded as high grade tumours irrespective of their grading.

Natural history

There is extensive local growth with infiltration of surrounding structures including blood vessels and nerves, and early blood-borne spread to lungs as the most common distant site.

Lymph node spread is relatively uncommon except for synovial sarcomas and alveolar rhabdomyosarcoma.

Symptoms

Peripheral sarcomas present as a lump which may be present for some time before it becomes symptomatic.

Retroperitoneal sarcomas may grow to a large size before causing symptoms, the most common of which is backache.

Rapid increase in size of a pre-existing neurofibroma should alert to the possibility of malignant change to a neurofibrosarcoma.

Signs

At presentation peripheral sarcomas are often large masses within soft tissue. Figure 15.1 demonstrates a large soft tissue sarcoma arising in the lower limb.

Movement can become limited particularly when close to joints. Retroperitoneal masses may be palpable per abdomen.

Differential diagnosis

Other benign soft tissue masses should be considered, such as a neurofibroma, lipoma or fibroma.

Investigations

Routine investigations such as full blood count and blood biochemistry are usually unremarkable.

Chest X-ray may show pulmonary metastases. If normal a CT scan of the chest should be performed to further exclude metastases.

CT scan or MRI of the primary site is valuable in defining the precise extent and involvement of local structures.

Biopsy of the primary lesion is essential to confirm the diagnosis and the type of sarcoma. Definition of a sarcoma may be difficult and if needle biopsy is not sufficient an open biopsy may be required. It is important that this is performed in consultation with the surgeon who will perform the definitive resection as implantation at the biopsy site can occur and this should be included in the resection.

Fig. 15.1   Soft tissue sarcoma (liposarcoma) of the lower limb.

Staging

Staging is based on the size of the primary tumour as follows:

T1 – Tumour < or = 5 cm max diameter.
T2 – Tumour > 5 cm max diameter.
N0 – No nodes.
N1 – Regional nodes.
G1 – Low grade.
G2 – Intermediate grade.
G3 – High grade.

Treatment

Local treatment

Wide surgical resection including excision of any previous biopsy scar, combined with radiotherapy which may be given pre- or post-operatively, enables conservation of the affected limb.

Amputation is avoided if at all possible.

Retroperitoneal tumours present a more difficult surgical problem and resection may not be possible. High dose irradiation is required delivering doses of at least 60 Gy in 6 weeks.

Radiation alone may control a soft tissue sarcoma but is inferior to the combination of surgery with irradiation.

Isolated limb perfusion with drugs such as melphelan may be of benefit in locally advanced, unresectable limb tumours.

Metastatic disease

Chemotherapy has only limited activity. Responses are seen with cisplatin, adriamycin and ifosphamide but long-term remissions are few and the toxicity of treatment is considerable.

Surgical resection (metastatectomy) is the most successful treatment of lung metastases if feasible.

Tumour-related complications

Local effects due to tumour size are the main problem associated with soft tissue sarcomas.

In general paraneoplastic effects and systemic complications such as hypercalcaemia are not features of these tumours, although hypoglycaemia has been described as a rare association with massive retroperitoneal sarcomas.

Treatment-related complications

The emphasis of modern treatment is towards limb preservation. However, the effects of extensive resection and radiotherapy may lead to functional deficits in the limb with joint stiffness, loss of muscle power and limb oedema.

Prognosis

The prognosis for peripheral limb tumours is better than that of sarcomas affecting the retroperitoneum, trunk or internal organs. With conservative limb-preserving treatment local control rates will be of the order of 80 per cent with 5 year survival around 60 per cent depending on the tumour stage and grade. Patients with operable lung metastases have a 5 year survival of around 30 per cent following metastatectomy.

Future developments

The major change in the management of soft tissue sarcomas has been in the development of limb-preserving treatment in the place of amputation. The main difficulty now lies in the management of systemic disease from which there is no satisfactory treatment. Adjuvant chemotherapy has been proposed as a possible way of reducing systemic relapse but trials to date have been disappointing.

Rare tumours

Desmoid tumours

These classically arise in the abdominal wall of women postpartum but in fact may occur at any site presenting as a diffuse fibrous infiltrative tumour which while pathologically benign may cause serious effects by virtue of its relentless local growth. Surgical resection is the treatment of choice but when inoperable slow regression is achieved following a radical dose of radiotherapy.

Stewart–Treves tumour

This is the name given to the rare development of a lymphangiosarcoma in the upper limb of a woman having chronic lymphoedema secondary to the treatment of breast carcinoma. Treatment may be difficult due to the pre-existing oedema and associated post-operative and post-radiotherapy changes. Amputation may be necessary.

Dermatofibroma

This is a benign tumour of the skin presenting as a fibrous nodule typically on the limbs, distinct from simple fibromas by the presence of histiocytes on microscopy. Its malignant counterpart is dermatofibrosarcoma protuberans, so called because of its microscopic appearance with an hour-glass shape pushing the epidermis outwards. Histologically it is essentially a fibrosarcoma and is usually found on the trunk.

Osteosarcoma

Epidemiology

Osteosarcoma is the most common malignant tumour of the bone although it is rare in relation to other malignancies. It occurs mainly in adolescents particularly during periods of active bone growth with a second peak of incidence in those over 60 years when it is related to Paget's disease. It is almost twice as common in males as females.

Aetiology

No recognizable aetiological agent is present for the majority of cases.

Paget's disease

May be a pre-existing feature in adult osteosarcoma, as shown in Figure 15.2.

Radiation

A rare late effect following therapeutic irradiation. Historically associated with radium dial painting and the use of thorotrast as contrast medium in diagnostic radiology.

Genetic

An association with the retinoblastoma gene with deletions on the long arm of chromosome 13 has been described.

(a)   (b)

Fig. 15.2 X-rays showing pre-existing Paget's disease of bone in a humerus (a) within which an osteosarcoma has subsequently developed (b).

Pathology

The most common site for osteosarcoma is in a long bone particularly around the knee, 30 per cent arising from the lower femur and 15 per cent in the upper tibia. Ten per cent arise in the humerus and the remainder may affect any bone including the axial skeleton.

Macroscopically the tumour arises in the metaphysis and grows both eccentrically, expanding the cortex and raising the periosteum at its edges, and also along the medulla. Within the tumour will be areas of haemorrhage and necrosis together with new bone formation in the subperiosteal regions to form the classical Codman's triangles and sunray spicules.

Pathological fracture through the tumour-bearing bone may occur.

Microscopically there are two main populations of cells: a background stroma of spindle-shaped sarcomatous cells containing a matrix which may be myxoid, cartilaginous or osteoid together with multinucleate giant cells.

Natural history

There is local spread within the bone of origin, typically within the medullary cavity, and early blood-borne spread particularly to the lungs. Other bones may also be affected through blood-borne spread.

Lymph node disease is not a prominent feature.

Symptoms

There is usually pain in the bone and there may be a lump around the site of origin. There is sometimes a history of preceding trauma although no causal relationship exists.

Symptoms from metastases may include cough and haemoptysis but other features of malignant disease such as anorexia and weight loss are infrequent unless very advanced.

Signs

Swelling and deformity of the bone. It is often hot and red and there may be an audible bruit. Thinning of the periosteum may result in a characteristic crackling on palpation and there may be crepitus if fracture has occurred.

There is often an associated fever.

Differential diagnosis

Other causes of bone swelling should be considered, including benign tumours such as osteochondromas and other malignant tumours.

Investigations

Routine investigations are often unremarkable although there may be a leucocytosis and the alkaline phosphatase will be inappropriately raised (remember that in growing children and adolescents the normal range for alkaline phosphatase is increased during bone growth).

Plain X-ray of the affected bone will show local destruction of bone with areas of new bone formation which may form the classical Codman's triangles and sunray spicules but more often are less well demarcated. There will be periosteal elevation and pathological fracture may be apparent. In adults co-existing Paget's disease may be apparent, as illustrated in Figure 15.2.

Further detail of the precise extent of bone destruction and spread within the medullary cavity will be found on CT or MRI scan.

CT scan of the lungs is important to identify pulmonary metastases.

Isotope bone scan will give further information on the extent of local bone involvement and also identify any bone metastases.

Staging

There is no widely used staging system for osteosarcoma.

Treatment

The mainstay of modern treatment for osteosarcoma is a course of intensive chemotherapy together with local removal or irradiation of the site of origin.

Chemotherapy

High dose methotrexate should be administered in doses of between 8 and 12 g/m² of body surface area. This involves intensive hydration schedules, urine alkalinization by the administration of oral sodium bicarbonate and the use of repeated doses of folinic acid 24 hours after the methotrexate to reverse residual systemic effects. Additional drugs are usually added to the schedule such as adriamycin, bleomycin, vincristine, cyclophosphamide and dactinomycin.

Recently simpler schedules have been designed based on the use of cisplatin, ifosphamide and adriamycin and these are being evaluated against the standard methotrexate-based schedules.

Local treatment

Following 6 to 8 weeks chemotherapy with satisfactory response conservative limb-preserving resection of the bone is undertaken. This may entail the use of an appropriate prosthesis or excision of the entire bone if expendable as in the case of a rib or the fibula.

For surgically unresectable disease local radiotherapy will be given with the aim of delivering a dose of up to 60 Gy in 6 weeks. In certain sites, particularly in the spine close to spinal cord, the dose may be limited by the tolerance of CNS tissue. Following local treatment chemotherapy will be continued for a total of around 20 weeks.

Metastases

Patients presenting with lung metastases will be treated in a similar fashion if resectable with metastatectomy being performed in addition to local surgery.

Palliation

Palliative treatment may be required for relapsed disease. Local irradiation may be valuable for local pain and to arrest tumour growth through skin. Amputation may be considered for recurrent disease but only when there is thought to be a realistic chance of long-term salvage.

Metastatic disease may require further chemotherapy and limited pulmonary metastases may be resected

Tumour-related complications

The principal complication is pathological fracture.

Treatment-related complications

The affected limb may have limitation of movement and muscle strength.

Prostheses fitted to young patients who have not completed their growth may require revision from time to time.

Following amputation which may still be required by a small number of patients specific problems may include phantom limb pain and stump ulceration and chafing.

Thoracotomy may result in limited respiratory reserve depending on the extent of resection required and post-operative pain in the thoracotomy scar is a well-recognized problem.

Chemotherapy will have considerable acute morbidity including nausea, vomiting, alopecia and mucositis. Longer-term problems may arise from nephrotoxicity related to the use of methotrexate or cisplatin and neurotoxicity from cisplatin or vincristine.

In children there may be growth retardation and effects on subsequent maturation and fertility.

Prognosis

Overall, using modern chemotherapy-based schedules for treatment, the 5 year survival for non-metastatic osteosarcoma is between 40 and 50 per cent. In patients presenting with lung metastases up to 20 per cent may become long- term survivors and as many as 40 per cent of those relapsing with pulmonary metastases may be salvaged.

Rare tumours

Parosteal sarcoma

This typically occurs in young adults arising from the juxtacortical part of the bone growing concentrically around the bone. The lower femur and upper tibia are the usual sites. Surgical excision is the treatment of choice. The prognosis is better than that for an osteosarcoma with 5 year survival figures of 50 to 70 per cent.

Ewing's sarcoma

Epidemiology

Ewing's sarcoma is a tumour of bone affecting predominantly children and young adults, the maximum incidence being between the ages of 10 and 20 years. A rare extra-osseous form of Ewing's is also recognized. The incidence of Ewing's in the UK is 0.6 in 100 000 and males are affected more than females. It is relatively rare in black populations.

Aetiology

There is no recognized aetiological agent but a specific chromosomal translocation in Ewing's has been demonstrated between chromosomes 11 and 22.

Pathology

Ewing's may affect any bone and is found in long bones, vertebrae and limb girdles, especially the pelvic bones. Macroscopically it arises in the diaphysis of the bone growing subperiosteally. Periosteal reaction as it traverses the length of the bone may give rise to the characteristic onion peel appearance of the bone on X-ray. To the naked eye the tumour contains areas of necrosis, and haemorrhage and cystic regions may also be seen.

Microscopically Ewing's is composed of sheets of small round cells which are rich in glycogen.

Natural history

There is local growth, the primary often reaching a considerable size, and blood-borne dissemination with metastases to lungs in particular.

Lymph node metastases are not usually a major feature.

Symptoms

Ewing's is typically painful and characteristically pain is intermittent in the early development of the tumour mass. There may be a preceding history of trauma but no causal relationship is recognized.

Pathological fracture may occur.

Lung metastases may cause cough or haemoptysis.

Signs

The tumour mass will be apparent as a palpable mass often tender to palpation. There may be associated fever particularly in advanced cases.

Differential diagnosis

Ewing's must be differentiated from other primary tumours of bone. Other round cell tumours which can affect bone should also be excluded, in particular lymphoma, neuroblastoma and anaplastic carcinoma.

Investigations

A full blood count may demonstrate a raised white cell count and occasionally a mild anaemia may also be present. Biochemical tests may be normal or show an inappropriately raised alkaline phosphatase.

X-ray of the affected bone will show thinning of the diaphysis and in later stages extensive bone destruction. The characteristic onion peel appearance of successive layers of periosteal reaction may also be seen.

CT scan or MRI will show greater detail of the tumour mass, in particular soft tissue invasion, and spread along the marrow cavity of the bone.

Chest X-ray and, if normal, CT scan of the lungs should be performed to evaluate the possibility of lung metastases.

Biopsy of the primary lesion is essential to confirm the diagnosis.

Staging

There is no recognised staging system for Ewing's sarcoma.

Treatment

Chemotherapy

The common chemotherapy schedule used is based on the use of VAC (vincristine, adriamycin and cyclophosphamide) and VCA (vincristine, cyclophosphamide and actinomycin D). Recently more intensive schedules based on ifosphamide, actinomycin D and adriamycin have been developed which may have even greater activity.

Local treatment

After 2 to 3 months of chemotherapy, radiotherapy will be the treatment of choice for most patients to deliver a total dose of between 50 and 60 Gy in 5 to 6 weeks.

Surgery may be used instead, particularly for bones such as rib and fibula which can be removed *in toto*.

Chemotherapy is then continued for several months following local treatment.

Palliative treatment

Standard chemotherapy as described above is appropriate for widespread symptomatic metastases. Local symptoms of pain or bleeding may be better dealt with by local radiotherapy. In selected patients high dose chemotherapy with autologous marrow transplant may be an option.

Tumour-related complications

- Pathological fracture.
- Spinal cord compression from rapid growth of spinal tumours.

Treatment-related complications

Chemotherapy may result in acute nausea, vomiting and alopecia. In the longer term vincristine can be associated with a peripheral neuropathy and in high doses adriamycin is cardiotoxic. For this reason it is spared by substituting actinomycin once a tolerance dose has been reached.

High dose radiotherapy to a limb may result in joint stiffness, skin changes and lymphoedema.

Prognosis

The overall 5 year survival for patients without metastases treated with modern chemotherapy-based regimes is around 50 per cent. This is determined particularly by tumour size ranging from 70 per cent in tumours less than 500 cc to 35 per cent in tumours greater than 500 cc.

Local control rates may approach 90 per cent and are greater in long bones than in the pelvis.

Other bone tumours

Chondrosarcoma

This is a tumour typically affecting the pelvic bones although it may also occur in the femur, humerus and scapula. It is a tumour of adults and usually slow growing. Rarely, they may arise within a pre-existing chondroma. Initial treatment is radical surgical resection or if inoperable radiotherapy. Well and moderately differentiated forms have a good prognosis and only metastasize late, if at all. There is, however, a high grade variant which has an aggressive course and these patients may be selected for treatment with early chemotherapy using drugs similar to the osteosarcoma schedules. The overall 5 year survival is around 35 per cent.

Osteoclastoma (giant cell tumour)

This is a tumour arising in adults usually between the ages of 30 and 50, the most common sites being the long bones around the knee, radius and humerus. There is a characteristic 'soap bubble' appearance on X-ray with eccentric thinning of the cortex. Clinically this may be demonstrated by 'egg shell crackling' on palpation.

It is composed of two populations of cells, a background stroma of spindle cells the differentiation of which defines the activity of the tumour and scattered multinucleate giant cells. The majority are of low grade malignancy and present a problem of local control rather than disseminated disease. Wide surgical excision is the treatment of choice. Around one-third will recur locally and a further one-third will be high grade tumours which ultimately metastasize. Local irradiation may be of value for local recurrence; chemotherapy is not usually successful in metastatic disease. The overall 5 year survival is around 65–70 per cent.

Spindle cell sarcoma

Tumours histologically identical to fibrosarcoma or malignant fibrous histiocytoma of soft tissue may be found as primary bone tumours. They are usually tumours of adults in the 30–60 age group. Treatment is radical surgical excision. There has been some interest in giving adjuvant chemotherapy in this group of patients but to date there is no evidence that this improves survival. Overall 5 year survivals are in the range 25–40 per cent.

Angiosarcomas may also arise in bone and will be treated in the same way as the other spindle cell sarcomas of bone.

16

Lymphoma

Malignancies of the lymphoproliferative system can be broadly classified into Hodgkin's disease and all other lymphomas which are termed the non-Hodgkin's lymphomas. The classification of these is complex and many different systems have been described. A simplified clinical view is shown in Figure 16.1.

Hodgkin's disease

Epidemiology

There are around 1300 cases per annum in the UK, with a bimodal age distribution – the two peaks of incidence occurring in young people aged 20–30 years and in later life between 60 and 70 years.

Overall it is almost twice as common in men as it is in women. In children the sex difference is even more extreme, occurring almost exclusively in boys under the age of 10 years.

It is rare in the Japanese and in the US black population, and particularly high in the Jewish populations of the US and the UK.

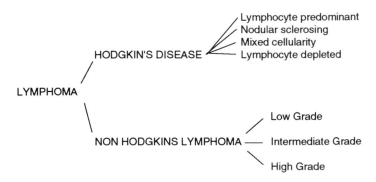

Fig. 16.1 Types of lymphoma.

Aetiology

There is no proven aetiological agent responsible for the development of Hodgkin's disease.

Pathology

Macroscopically Hodgkin's disease is usually found in lymph nodes, the spleen and liver. More rarely infiltration of the lungs, bone marrow, skin or central nervous system may occur. Typically the nodes are relatively soft and uniformly enlarged. The spleen and liver appearances are of multiple nodules within their substance, the cut surface of which has been likened to that of a German sausage.

Microscopically the diagnostic feature is the presence of binucleate cells called Reed–Sternberg cells. In addition a wide variation of other cells including lymphocytes, neutrophils, plasma cells, eosinophils, histiocytes and fibroblasts are also found infiltrating the node or affected organ. There are four major histological subclassifications, as shown in Table 16.1.

Table 16.1   Histological subtypes of Hodgkin's disease

Subclass	Features	Prognosis
Lymphocyte predominant	Infiltrate of many small lymphocytes	Good
Nodular sclerosis	Node divided by fibrous bands. Cells may be rich in lymphocytes (type 1) or be of mixed type (type 2)	Type 1 – good Type 2 – moderate
Mixed cellularity	Mixed population of cells	Moderate
Lymphocyte depleted	Fibrous node with Reed–Sternberg cells but few other cells seen	Poor

Natural history

Typically stepwise involvement of adjacent node groups occurs. The most common nodes involved are those in the neck. In this situation spread is to adjacent nodes in the supraclavicular fossa, the axillae and the mediastinum before involving para-aortic nodes below the diaphragm. Extranodal involvement as a sole manifestation is rare and usually occurs in the context of extensive or bulky node disease.

Symptoms

Typically the patient is aware of a painless enlarged node in the neck. This may be present for many weeks or months but may develop more rapidly.
   'B' symptoms are characteristic of lymphomas and are:

- Fever greater than 38° often with typical remittant pattern (Pel–Ebstein fever).
- Weight loss of more than 10 per cent body weight.
- Night sweats.

   Other symptoms include:

- Generalized and often intractable itching.
- Alcohol-induced pain in the enlarged nodes.
- Although the lymph nodes themselves are usually painless there may be back ache from para-aortic nodes and left-sided abdominal pain from splenic enlargement.

Signs

Enlarged lymph nodes may be present in any site. They are most common in the neck. Typically the nodes of Hodgkin's disease are described as firm and rubbery as opposed to the hard craggy nodes of carcinoma.
   There may be palpable hepatosplenomegaly or an abdominal mass due to para-aortic or mesenteric nodes.
   Inguinal and pelvic lymphadenopathy may be associated with oedema of the lower limbs although arm oedema is an unusual complication of axillary lymphadenopathy. Mediastinal lymphadenopathy may present with the signs of superior vena cava obstruction.

Differential diagnosis

The main differential diagnosis will be to distinguish Hodgkin's from non-Hodgkin's lymphoma.
   Other causes of lymphadenopathy will also be considered including infection which can be either pyogenic, tuberculous or viral, e.g. EB or CMV viruses, toxoplasmosis and other neoplastic conditions such as leukaemia or carcinoma.

Investigations

A full blood count may show mild anaemia and leucocytosis with a raised lymphocyte count but is frequently normal.
   ESR may be raised, particularly in more aggressive forms of the disease.
   Routine biochemical blood tests may show evidence of hepatic infiltration with raised alkaline phosphatase and gammaglutamyltransferase. More profound hepatic disturbance is rare. Obstruction of the renal tracts by enlarged nodes may cause renal failure. Hypercalcaemia is a recognised but rare finding in Hodgkin's disease.

Serum lactate dehydrogenase is a sensitive index of disease activity and of prognostic importance.

Bone marrow aspirate and trephine should be examined for evidence of infiltration with Hodgkin's disease.

Chest X-ray may show widened mediastinal shadow due to enlarged nodes or, more rarely, lung parenchymal infiltration. Pleural effusion is also a recognized finding.

CT scan of the chest, abdomen and pelvis will give the most accurate assessment of internal lymphadenopathy and has now superseded the use of bipedal lymphangiography as the imaging of choice for staging in lymphoma.

A tissue diagnosis is mandatory to confirm the diagnosis and define the histological subtype of Hodgkin's disease. This will usually take the form of an open lymph node biopsy from an accessible node in the neck, supraclavicular fossa or groin.

Splenectomy was in the past a standard procedure to complete the staging of Hodgkin's disease. It is now performed only rarely since current indications for systemic treatment mean that information about splenic status will rarely influence management, and imaging with ultrasound, CT and MRI will give an accurate picture of subdiaphragmatic disease for which previously laparotomy was required.

Staging

The staging of Hodgkin's disease follows the Ann Arbor classification, as shown in Table 16.2.

Table 16.2 Staging of Hodgkin's disease

Stage 1	Involved lymph nodes limited to one node area only
Stage 2	Involved lymph nodes involving two or more adjacent areas but remaining on one side of the diaphragm only
Stage 3	Involved lymph nodes on both sides of the diaphragm
Stage 4	Involvement of extranodal organs denoted by the following suffixes:
	M – bone marrow
	D – skin
	H – liver
	S – spleen

Each stage is further subclassified 'a' or 'b' according to the absence or presence respectively of 'b' symptoms (see above).

Treatment

Hodgkin's disease is both radiosensitive and chemosensitive and most patients can expect to be cured of their disease. Because this is a disease frequently affecting young people who will live for many years after successful treatment, there is now considerable emphasis not only on the efficacy of treatment but also on achieving cure with minimal long-term morbidity.

Localized disease (stages 1a and 2a)

Radical radiotherapy alone will cure many patients. This may take the form of 'involved field' irradiation where a volume including only those areas known to be affected is treated, or wide field irradiation. The former approach is associated with a greater chance of regional relapse but with less morbidity. Relapse in these patients can in most cases be salvaged using chemotherapy.

The usual radiotherapy fields treated are a 'mantle' field above the diaphragm and an inverted 'Y' below the diaphragm. These are shown in Figure 16.2.

Hodgkin's disease is very much more sensitive to radiation than the common epithelial cancers and requires only 35 to 40 Gy given over 4 to 4.5 weeks.

Advanced disease (stages 1b, 2b, 3 and 4)

Although there may be only limited nodal disease apparent the presence of 'b' symptoms is a poor prognostic feature and implies more widespread disease. For this reason stages 1b and 2b disease are included in this category together with those patients who have widespread node disease or involvement of systemic organs. Chemotherapy is given to these patients.

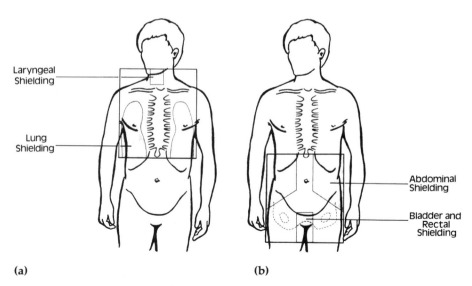

(a)   (b)

Fig. 16.2 Radiation fields for the treatment of Hodgkin's disease: (a) 'mantle' fields for nodes above the diaphragm; and (b) inverted 'Y' field for nodes below the diaphragm.

Prior to starting chemotherapy male patients should have the opportunity to consider sperm banking as subsequent fertility cannot be guaranteed after chemotherapy.

All patients having chemotherapy should be well hydrated and started on allopurinol to prevent tumour lysis syndrome (see Chapter 22).

Response may be dramatic and rapid; an example of a chemotherapy response on treating bulky mediastinal nodes from Hodgkin's disease is shown in Figure 16.3.

Specific chemotherapy

Early schedules used were based upon MOPP (mustine, vincristine, procarbazine and prednisolone). While effective in giving complete remission rates of up to 80 per cent there is significant toxicity and modifications have been developed to minimize this morbidity.

LOPP or ChlVPP replaces the mustine by chlorambucil and in the case of ChlVPP, vincristine is replaced by vinblastine.

Anthracycline-based (i.e. adriamycin or its analogues) schedules such as ABVD (adriamycin, bleomycin, vincristine and DTIC) are also highly active and are now often used alternating with LOPP/ChlVPP. They are associated with less long-term toxicity.

Most patients will receive six courses of chemotherapy.

Radiotherapy is then usually given following (or sometimes in the middle of) chemotherapy, except for those patients with stage 4 disease affecting major organs or bone marrow.

Treatment for relapse

Relapse after radiotherapy will generally be treated with chemotherapy and response rates similar to other patients receiving primary chemotherapy are to be expected with around 80 per cent going back into remission.

Relapse after chemotherapy is not so easy to treat. Of those patients given initial chemotherapy for advanced disease around 40 per cent will either relapse or fail to achieve a sustained complete remission. Retreatment with the same or alternative chemotherapy regimes may result in further regression of disease for around 50 per cent but

Fig. 16.3 Chest X-ray before and after chemotherapy for extensive mediastinal Hodgkin's disease.

of these only 15–20 per cent will achieve long-term remission. It is therefore in this group of patients that more intensive treatment using high dose chemotherapy and bone marrow autograft may be indicated. With such techniques long-term survival may be achieved in over 30 per cent of patients relapsing after conventional chemotherapy for Hodgkin's disease.

Tumour-related complications

Massive lymphadenopathy may have consequences as a result of local pressure, although in general lymphoma tends to grow around structures rather than directly invade them. In the mediastinum dysphagia and superior vena cava obstruction may occur. In the abdomen renal failure due to ureteric obstruction and lower limb oedema due to pelvic node enlargement are seen.

Treatment-related complications

Radiotherapy

Wide field irradiation may have various long-term effects although it should be emphasized that for most patients there are few if any sequelae. The potential problems are shown in Table 16.3.

Table 16.3   Late effects of radiotherapy for Hodgkin's disease

Site	Late radiation effects
Neck	Hypothyroidism. Treatment in puberty may induce thyroid cancer, loss of muscle and soft tissue bulk causing asymmetry
Mediastinum	Pneumonitis and lung fibrosis. Pericarditis
Spinal cord	Myelitis
Abdomen	Increased incidence of peptic ulceration
Pelvis	Amenorrhoea in women and sterility if gonads included in radiation field

Chemotherapy

Acute toxicity includes nausea and vomiting, alopecia and bone marrow depression. Neutropenic sepsis is a potential hazard of any such treatment. Peripheral neuropathy may develop from the use of vincristine or less commonly vinblastine.

Adriamycin has specific dose-related cardiotoxic effects and bleomycin may cause lung damage at high doses. Neither of these effects will be expected in standard treatment schedules but may become a potential hazard in patients requiring retreatment.

The anthracycline-containing schedules such as ABVD have the advantage of preserving fertility whereas after MOPP-type regimes most patients are sterile, men being more sensitive than women.

There is increasing concern regarding the incidence of second malignancies in patients who are cured of their Hodgkin's disease. There is an ongoing risk with time from treatment which appears to be rising to over 15 per cent in patients who have survived for 20 years or more. In the early years occasional leukaemias or non-Hodgkin's lymphomas are diagnosed but the major problem appears to be an increasing risk of solid tumours as the years pass.

The exact cause for this remains unclear. The greatest incidence is in those patients receiving both radiotherapy and chemotherapy while the risk for patients receiving radiotherapy alone appears negligible. It is thought that the newer anthracyclin-containing schedules may be safer in this respect. The influence of the disease itself in this phenomenon is also unclear.

Prognosis

Overall the prognosis for patients diagnosed with Hodgkin's disease is good. Virtually all patients presenting with stage 1a disease will be cured and 50–60 per cent of those with advanced disease (stages 3b or 4) may also expect cure.

Future prospects

Increasingly the emphasis in Hodgkin's disease now is to maintain the very high cure rates obtained while reducing morbidity. This is achieved by developing new, less toxic chemotherapy schedules and reducing the routine use of radiotherapy. Lower doses of radiation may also be adequate particularly in combination with chemotherapy.

For those patients with advanced disease who relapse or fail to achieve remission there is increasing use of high dose salvage treatment with or without bone marrow transplantation.

Non-Hodgkin's lymphoma (NHL)

Epidemiology

There are around 5000 cases of non-Hodgkin's lymphoma in the UK each year, accounting for 2 per cent of all maligancies. It occurs equally in men and women and the incidence increases with age, being relatively unusual under the age of 50. As with Hodgkin's disease there is a marked low incidence in the Japanese and American black population.

Aetiology

No single aetiological agent has been identified to account for the common forms of lymphoma found in the UK.

Infective agents

These include:

- EB virus associated with Burket's lymphoma found predominantly in Africa.
- HTLV type 1 virus associated with T-cell lymphoma found in the Caribbean and Japan.
- HIV infection is also associated with an excess of lymphomas and is probably a feature of their immunosuppressed status rather than a direct causation by virus.

Altered immune status

In addition to HIV NHL is also increased in other disease states associated with a depressed immune system including rheumatoid arthritis, coeliac disease, hypogammaglobulinaemia and following iatrogenic immune suppression after renal transplantation.

There are also associations with autoimmune disease such as Hashimoto's thyroiditis and thyroid lymphoma and Sjogren's disease and salivary gland lymphoma.

Irradiation

This may also be a factor in the development of NHL and increased incidences are seen following exposure in Hiroshima and Nagasaki, and after low dose therapeutic irradiation to the spine for ankylosing spondylitis.

Pathology

NHL describes a spectrum of neoplastic conditions as a result of which many complex and confusing classifications have arisen. The majority of NHL arise from the B lymphocyte but there is a well-recognized group which are undoubtedly T-cell derived neoplasms. Rare forms of histiocytic neoplasm also occur.

Macroscopically NHL will occur as a mass of neoplastic lymphoid tissue which may reach a considerable size. Ulceration, necrosis and haemorrhage are unusual. It may arise in recognized lymph node chains but, unlike Hodgkin's disease, extranodal lymphoma is relatively common with up to 50 per cent involving sites such as Waldeyer's ring, the gastrointestinal tract, skin and bone.

Microscopically the appearances are complex and interpretation can be difficult. In broad terms lymphomas may be low grade or high grade. Features of low grade lymphoma are the preservation of follicular

architecture and cellular composition of well-differentiated small lymphocytes. In contrast, high grade lymphomas are characterized by diffuse
infiltration of the gland or extranodal site with large undifferentiated
lymphoid cells. Some classifications, notably that of the National Cancer
Institute of the United States have introduced an intermediate category
and this Working Formulation is probably the most widely used currently.
The principles of its classification are shown in Table 16.4.

Table 16.4 Simplified classification of non-Hodgkin's lymphoma

Low grade (40%)
Well differentiated
Follicular lymphoma with any of the following cell types:
Lymphocytic lymphoma
   small cleaved cells
   mixed small cleaved and large cells
Intermediate grade (40%)
Follicular lymphoma containing predominantly large cells
Diffuse lymphoma containing any of the following cell types:
   small cleaved cells
   mixed small and large cells
   predominantly large cells
High grade (20%)
Immunoblastic
Lymphoblastic
Small non-cleaved cell as in Burket's lymphoma
Unclassified
Mycosis fungoides
True histiocytic lymphomas
Extramedullary plasmacytoma

The histological diagnosis of lymphoma is now supported by a range
of specific monoclonal antibody stains. Distinction from a poorly differentiated small cell carcinoma is made using the leucocyte common
antigen (LCA). Distinction of one subtype of lymphocyte from another
has become a complex science. Monoclonal antibody stains are applied
to frozen sections of biopsied material to differentiate B cells from T cells
from histiocytes and a large library of stains has now been built up to enable
subtyping of any lymphoma.

Natural history

Low grade lymphoma may be very indolent, remaining asymptomatic for
many years and, in the elderly, having little impact upon their life expectancy.

A high grade immunoblastic or lymphoblastic lymphoma is an aggressive often rapidly fatal condition.

Extranodal lymphoma may have a relatively benign course as in a low
grade skin lymphoma existing as purplish nodules requiring little else than
gentle local treatment from time to time, or an aggressive course as in a

high grade lymphoma of the bowel or central nervous system.

In general NHL unlike Hodgkin's disease does not have a clear pattern of contiguous spread from one area to the next. Dissemination is often wide and unpredictable following a pattern closer to that of a carcinoma with frequent hepatic and lung involvement.

Symptoms

Usually presents with a painless lump in a lymph node area, most commonly the neck but also the axilla or groin. There may be backache due to enlarged para-aortic nodes or upper abdominal pain from hepatosplenomegaly.

'B' symptoms as described for Hodgkin's disease are also an important feature – namely weight loss, fever and night sweats.

Other symptoms relate to the site of origin of an extranodal lymphoma.

NHL arising in Waldeyer's ring therefore will cause local symptoms similar to those of a carcinoma in these regions, with local pain or discomfort and epistaxis or nasal discharge where the nasopharynx is involved.

Gastointestinal lymphoma usually presents with an acute abdominal event due to haemorrhage, perforation or obstruction.

CNS lymphoma may cause symptoms of raised intracranial pressure with headache, vomiting and fits. Focal neurological features may cause bulbar palsy, diplopia, limb weakness and altered sensation.

Skin lymphoma usually presents as asymptomatic lumps but mycosis fungoides has a characteristic pre-tumour phase often lasting many years with chronic skin change which may be itchy and resemble dermatitis in its clinical picture.

Signs

Enlarged lymph nodes will be palpable, typically painless, firm, 'rubbery' nodes clinically indistinguishable from those of Hodgkin's disease but different from the hard craggy nodes of carcinoma.

At extranodal sites lymphoma often has a characteristic purplish appearance stretching overlying surfaces and ulcerating only rarely.

Hepatosplenomegaly is a common finding in both nodal and extranodal lymphoma.

Investigations

A full blood count may show signs of mild anaemia or pancytopenia if there is bone marrow involvement. A high white count composed predominantly of lymphocytes may also be found and is a relatively poor prognostic sign.

The ESR will be raised; an ESR greater than 40 mm/h is a further poor prognostic feature.

Routine biochemistry may show signs of hepatic infiltration. Renal failure is an infrequent complication of massive para-aortic node enlargement causing ureteric obstruction. The serum lactate dehydrogenase

(LDH) is a marker of disease activity.

The chest X-ray may show mediastinal lymphadenopathy or more rarely infiltration of the lung parenchyma.

Imaging of the abdominal and pelvic lymph nodes is best performed using a CT scan which has now superseded the use of bipedal lymphangiography.

Bone marrow examination will be required to assess the possibility of marrow infiltration.

Other imaging may be indicated depending on the site of origin. For bowel lymphoma a full barium series is performed since multiple foci of disease are well recognized. A CT scan of the brain will be performed for CNS lymphoma which may be further supplemented by an MRI scan to image potential spinal disease.

A CSF examination for lymphoma cells will be required for CNS lymphoma and may also be considered for other types considered to have a high risk CNS involvement, in particular diffuse large cell and lymphoblastic lymphomas.

Differential diagnosis

The main differential diagnosis rests between NHL and Hodgkin's disease. Epithelial tumours may be considered where NHL arises in extranodal sites. It may be difficult to distinguish clinically a low grade lymphoma with extensive bone marrow involvement from chronic lymphocytic leukaemia and lymphoblastic lymphoma from acute lymphoblastic leukaemia.

Staging

The Ann Arbor staging system is used for NHL as for Hodgkin's disease (see Table 16.2) with the further addition of a suffix 'E' where the lymphoma has arisen in an extranodal site. For example, a NHL arising in the tonsil with involved nodes in the neck would be stage 2 by virtue of the presence of two or more sites all on the same side of the diaphragm and be designated stage 2E, having arisen in an extranodal site.

Treatment

Treatment is based on histological grade and stage.

Low grade NHL

This is a condition which is rarely curable but usually has a long indolent course.

Localized low grade NHL (stage 1A) – local radiotherapy

- The involved area only is treated.
- A dose of 40 Gy in 4 weeks is usually given.

Other stages

Treated only when symptomatic using single agent oral chemotherapy of which the most popular is chlorambucil. There is no advantage to adding other drugs to chlorambucil in this setting. Alternatively single agent cyclophosphamide may be used and 70–80 per cent of patients will enter remission with either agent.

Relapse

Low grade lymphoma which is not localized is never cured, although survival for many years is to be expected. At some point, however, relapse is inevitable.

Retreatment with chlorambucil is often successful and local sites causing symptoms can be irradiated.

Patients who fail to respond to chlorambucil are usually treated more aggressively using combination chemotherapy such as CHOP in the same way that a high grade lymphoma will be treated (see below).

Transformation

Richter's syndrome refers to the transformation from a low grade to a high grade lymphoma which may occur in up to 15 per cent of patients presenting initially with low grade lymphoma. For this reason re-biopsy of recurrent disease should be considered before treatment.

Palliation

Steroids alone in moderate doses (40–60 mg of prednisolone) may have a valuable anti-tumour effect as well as their general effects in improving appetite and general well-being.

Single agent etoposide or vincristine may be used for subsequent relapses. Hemi-body irradiation is a valuable palliative treatment for widespread NHL no longer responsive to chemotherapy.

Intermediate/high grade lymphoma

This is a much more aggressive condition than low grade lymphoma and in general requires more intensive therapy.

Nodal lymphoma

Localized high grade NHL (stages 1A and 1E) – less than 10 per cent

- Local radiotherapy to affected area only.
- Chemotherapy is sometimes given in addition to local irradiation but its role in early lymphoma is unproven.

Advanced disease (stage 1B, 2, 3 or 4)

- Chemotherapy.

As for Hodgkin's disease consideration should be given to sperm banking for young males and all patients should be maintained well-hydrated and started on allopurinol to prevent tumour lysis syndrome (see Chapter 22).

Specific chemotherapy

Usually combination chemotherapy is given of which the most widely used is CHOP (Cyclophosphamide, adriamycin (Hydroxydaunorubicin), vincristine (Oncovin) and (Prednisolone). This is given as injections of the first three drugs on days 1 and 8 of a 28 day cycle with oral steroids on the first 8 days. A total of six courses is usually given.

Alternative schedules give weekly drugs over a 12 week course. These cycles are in general associated with greater toxicity, in particular neutropenia with the risk of sepsis and mucositis, and offer no advantage over standard chemotherapy in terms of patient survival.

Combined modality treatment

Sites of original bulky disease are often irradiated on the basis that these are frequently the sites of initial relapse. There is no good evidence that this practice significantly improves survival particularly in those patients who achieve a complete response to chemotherapy.

Lymphoblastic lymphoma

This form of high grade lymphoma has a particularly aggressive course and resembles acute lymphoblastic leukaemia in many of its features, for example a propensity to spread to the CNS. Results from standard lymphoma chemotherapy as described above are poor and most of these patients will be treated in protocols similar to those for ALL, including CNS prophylaxis.

Extranodal lymphoma

In general these lymphoma, are intermediate grade and will be treated in the same way as lymphomas arising in nodes as described above. There are, however, certain features of management particular to specific sites.

Waldeyer's ring lymphomas

Usually arise in the tonsils or nasopharynx. If early and non-bulky radiotherapy alone may be used including the whole of Waldeyer's ring in the treatment volume. More advanced disease will receive four to six courses of chemotherapy, e.g. CHOP followed by irradiation.

Gastrointestinal tract lymphomas

Often present as a surgical emergency and proceed to laparotomy at which bowel resection is performed. The diagnosis of NHL having been made these patients will be treated with chemotherapy. A well-recognized hazard of initial chemotherapy in these patients is that of intestinal perforation as the lymphoma in the bowel wall regresses and careful observation as an inpatient is usually recommended for the first course of treatment. Irradiation is difficult in these patients as it is difficult to demarcate clearly the affected area using standard localization techniques and the bowel tolerates irradiation poorly.

Skin lymphomas

Often low grade (lymphoma cutis) and require only gentle local treatment from time to time.

Mycosis fungoides is a characteristic T-cell skin lymphoma which has a long pre-tumour phase before developing into the characteristic skin infiltration which may be widespread. It responds poorly to chemotherapy. Less severe forms may respond to PUVA (psoralens and ultraviolet A exposure) and for others local irradiation is required. In widespread disease the entire body may be affected when irradiation of the whole body with electrons will be required.

CNS lymphoma

This has a poor prognosis. It has a propensity to seed throughout the central nervous system via the CSF circulation. Conventional treatment includes irradiation of the entire CNS axis from the cerebral hemispheres to the sacral region but this has only limited success. There is some suggestion that adding chemotherapy to this may improve results but most patients will still relapse after only a relatively short time.

Primary lymphoma of bone

May, if still localized to the bone of origin, be cured by local radiotherapy alone. Conventionally the entire bone is included in the radiation field. More extensive disease will require the addition of chemotherapy.

Bone marrow transplantation in NHL

Although not part of the current first line management of NHL, high dose chemotherapy with or without total body irradiation and either autograft or allograft is increasingly being considered for patients with intermediate and high grade lymphomas who relapse after initial response to chemotherapy. Up to a third of selected patients may be cured after relapse using this approach.

Tumour-related complications

Given the great heterogeneity of NHL a vast range of clinical complications may arise, most of which have been covered in the above text.

Mass effects from malignant nodes or lymphomatous tissue compromising normal function so that, for example, mediastinal disease may cause SVC obstruction or dysphagia, abdominal disease may cause renal failure due to ureteric obstruction, pelvic disease may cause oedema of the lower limbs.

Gastrointestinal lymphoma may cause bowel haemorrhage, obstruction or perforation.

CNS lymphoma may cause focal neurological damage or obstructive hydrocephalus.

Treatment-related complications

Radiotherapy

Late toxicity related to site, e.g. irradiating Waldeyer's ring, may cause dry mouth, taste loss and dental problems. Abdominal and pelvic irradiation may result in post-radiation bowel and bladder changes.

Chemotherapy

During treatment bone marrow depression, with the risks of neutropenic sepsis, occurs together with nausea, vomiting, alopecia and mucositis.

In the longer term adriamycin may cause dose-related cardiotoxicity, and bleomycin is associated with dose-related pneumonitis and lung fibrosis together with peripheral skin changes.

Second malignancy in patients with NHL is becoming more apparent as the results of treatment improve and more patients survive to develop a new malignancy. It is estimated that the risk of developing acute myeloblastic leukaemia in the first 5 years following treatment is between 6 and 8 per cent and as with Hodgkin's disease appears most marked in patients treated with both chemotherapy and radiotherapy. There is a less clear association with the development of solid tumours (i.e. cancers or sarcomas) as yet but since it is known that this risk increases with time over 20 or 30 years it is likely to emerge as cohorts if cured patients are followed for this length of time.

Prognosis

The prognosis for low grade lymphoma is better than intermediate or high grade lymphomas with median survival of 8–10 years reported from most centres.

Intermediate grade localized lymphoma will be cured by local radiotherapy in around 80 per cent of patients. Extranodal lymphoma, even when localized, tends to have a worse prognosis than nodal lymphoma; Waldeyer's ring and skin do better than gastrointestinal tract which does better than CNS.

More advanced intermediate and high grade NHL will respond to chemotherapy in most patients with complete regression of disease in

70–80 per cent, however long-term survival figures tend to fall below 50 per cent at 5 years from treatment.

Future prospects

The main areas of development in the management of NHL are concerned with defining the place of high dose chemotherapy with bone marrow or peripheral stem cell autograft for those patients requiring intensive therapy. There are new anti-lymphocytic drugs such as fludarabine currently being evaluated in low grade lymphoma and attempts are being made to use less toxic combination chemotherapy schedules in more aggressive lymphomas, particularly in the elderly who tolerate such treatment poorly and have much higher treatment-related morbidity and mortality.

Rare tumours

Malignant histiocytosis

A rare form of lymphoma characterized by systemic symptoms of fever, weight loss, generalized lymphadenopathy, hepatosplenomegaly and pancytopaenia. Histiocytic lymphoma is typically associated with coeliac disease when it presents as a multicentric bowel lymphoma. It may respond to lymphoma-type chemotherapy but the prognosis is generally much worse than other forms of lymphoma.

Castleman's disease

Probably not a neoplasm but a hamartomatous condition of lymphoid tissue. It may present in a similar fashion to lymphoma and histological differentiation can be difficult. It is uncertain whether active treatment other than simple excision of affected nodes is of value although there are reports of successful regression after irradiation.

17

Haematological malignancy

Leukaemia

Neoplastic conditions of the haemopoetic and lymphoid systems are closely related. Subclassifications of leukaemias and lymphomas tend to be complex but clinical management is usually based on a more simple and pragmatic division of leukaemias into acute or chronic, lymphoid or myeloid.

There are around 4800 cases of leukaemias registered per year in the UK and these account for around 4000 deaths each year.

Acute leukaemia

Acute leukaemia may be subclassified by its cell of origin into two broad groups: lymphoblastic and myeloblastic.

Acute lymphoblastic leukaemia (ALL)

Epidemiology

ALL is less common than acute myeloid leukaemia, affecting males and females in equal proportions. It is predominantly a malignancy affecting children with 40 per cent occurring in the 3 to 5 year old age group when it predominates in boys.

Aetiology

Down's syndrome is associated with a higher incidence.

Environmental agents, e.g. viruses: clustering of cases in certain areas of the UK has been described but it is uncertain whether this is related to any specific environmental agent.

Chromosomal translocations have been identified which are thought to activate the oncogene c-myc following translocation of its sequence from chromosome 8 where it normally resides.

Radiation exposure may be implicated, although post-radiation leukaemia is usually myeloblastic.

Pathology

Lymphoblastic leukaemia is characterized by the presence of large immature lymphoblasts throughout the reticuloendothelial system. These cells are distinguished from other cells such as myeloblasts by their staining, as shown in Table 17.1.

ALL is also subclassified according to the type of lymphoid cell which has become neoplastic and by the cell morphology, as shown in Table 17.2.

In addition to *de novo* ALL up to 15 per cent of cases represent transformation into an acute phase from chronic myeloid leukaemia (CML). These are characterized by possessing the Philadelphia chromosome (see below).

Natural history

Progressive infiltration of the bone marrow and subsequent bone marrow failure ensues. It may also affect other sites, in particular the CNS where diffuse meningeal infiltration may be seen and in males the testes.

Symptoms

Patients present with bone marrow failure which results in: malaise, lethargy, effort dyspnoea or angina due to progressive anaemia; infection due to leucopenia; and bleeding in the form of epistaxis, haematuria or haemoptysis due to thrombocytopenia.

Table 17.1   Staining characteristics of ALL compared with AML

	PAS	TdT	Sudan Black
ALL	+	+	−
AML	−	−	+

PAS = periodic acid Schiff. TdT = terminal deoxynucleotidyl transferase.

Table 17.2   Subclassification of ALL

Morphological

L1	L2	L3
Small uniform blast cells with high nuclear/cytoplasmic ratio	Larger blast cells lower nuclear/ cytoplasmic ratio	Vacuolated blasts basophilic cytoplasm

Cell type

	Surface Ig	Rosette formation	Proportion
B cell	+	−	2%
T cell	−	+	15%
Common	+	+	75%
Null	−	−	8%

Bone pains may also be present.

There are also general symptoms of malignancy including fever, sweats and weight loss.

Signs

- Peripheral lymphadenopathy is common.
- Splenomegaly.
- The liver may also be palpable.
- Purpura may be apparent particularly on the lower limbs as may other signs of recent haemorrhage from the nose or oral cavity.
- Signs of infection with fever and oropharyngeal or chest signs.

Differential diagnosis

Other types of acute leukaemia or high grade non-Hodgkin's lymphoma should be considered.

Other causes of pancytopenia must also be considered including aplastic anaemia.

Infection with Epstein–Barr (EB) virus may give a similar picture with abnormal blast cells seen in the peripheral blood.

Investigations

A full blood count will show pancytopenia. The blood film will reveal the presence of lymphoblasts.

The ESR will be raised.

Liver function tests may be abnormal.

Chest X-ray may show evidence of leukaemic infiltration or more commonly infection. A mediastinal mass of lymph nodes may be demonstrated.

A bone marrow aspirate and trephine is required to confirm the diagnosis with an excess of abnormal lymphoblasts. Specific stains will then be applied to subtype the cells into common, T, B or null ALL.

Staging

There is no formal staging system for the leukaemias. However, the important features which determine prognosis are:

- Subtype, common ALL having a good prognosis.
- Total white blood cell count, a total count of more than 20 000 being associated with a poor prognosis.

Other favourable features are female sex, young age and the absence of a mediastinal mass.

Treatment

The treatment of acute leukaemias can be considered in three phases: induction, consolidation and maintenance. Alongside this intensive supportive treatment may be necessary using blood products and antibiotics. In the UK most centres will treat patients within the national UKALL protocols through which modifications to treatment schedules have been tested in prospective randomized studies.

Induction

Using vincristine and prednisolone with the addition of other agents such as adriamycin, daunorubicin or l-asparaginase this can improve response rates from 50 per cent with vincristine and prednisolone alone to around 70 per cent. Induction therapy will usually continue over a period of 8 weeks.

Consolidation

This may be necessary once remission is achieved, i.e. when abnormal leukaemic cells are no longer detectable in the peripheral blood and bone marrow. This will take the form of prophylactic treatment to the CNS using radiotherapy to the whole brain and intrathecal injections of methotrexate.

Maintenance

Chemotherapy will then be given with methotrexate and mercaptopurine which may be continued for a total of 2 to 3 years.

Bone marrow transplantation

Increasingly high dose chemotherapy with bone marrow transplantation is being considered for poor risk patients who achieve initial remission. This is particularly the case for adults who have a much worse prognosis from ALL than children, especially those with Philadelphia chromosome present on the leukaemic cells. Bone marrow transplantation is also indicated for children who relapse with bone marrow disease after initial chemotherapy.

Bone marrow transplantation is an intensive treatment which involves exposure of the patient to very high doses of chemotherapy, usually cyclophosphamide or melphelan and whole body irradiation. This has the effect of completely ablating the bone marrow which then has to be replaced. This may be from a matched donor (allograft) or from the patient's marrow previously collected and stored while in remission (autograft). The patient's marrow may be treated with monoclonal antibody techniques in an attempt to purge it further of residual leukaemic cells.

Intensive support is required for the period from marrow ablation to the re-establishment of the grafted marrow, which may be 3 to 4 weeks. During this time blood and platelet transfusions are required. Antibiotic prophylaxis is given with aggressive treatment of any febrile episode using high dose broad spectrum antibiotics for bacterial, viral and fungal infections. Despite this even in experienced units a mortality rate of around 5 per cent may be expected from the procedure usually due to neutropenic infection or pneumonitis. Mortality is in general related to age and bone marrow transplantation is a hazardous undertaking in patients over the age of 50 years.

A further complication of allograft bone marrow transplantation is that of graft versus host disease in which the graft marrow reacts against the host tissues. This may manifest itself in a number of ways most commonly through hepatic dysfunction, gastrointestinal disturbance and skin rashes. Various attempts have been made to reduce this event by treating the donor marrow to remove T lymphocytes which are the principal cell type involved and by the use of immunosuppressive agents such as methotrexate or azathioprine.

Relapse treatment

When ALL has failed to respond to first line chemotherapy or has relapsed following initial treatment. The usual pattern of relapse is with bone marrow disease. CNS relapse occurs in up to 10 per cent of cases despite CNS prophylaxis and will require treatment with local irradiation and intrathecal therapy. Testicular relapse will be treated with local irradiation.

Salvage chemotherapy may take the form of using standard induction chemotherapy as above with alternative drugs added such as cytosine arabinoside. For those with a matched donor available then bone marrow transplant is indicated.

Tumour-related complications

Pancytopenia with consequent anaemia, leucopenia predisposing to infection and thrombocytopenia-related haemorrhage may occur.

Treatment-related complications

Tumour lysis syndrome is a rare complication arising as a result of the breakdown of large numbers of lymphoid cells when chemotherapy is initiated. This is discussed in full in Chapter 22.

Bone marrow suppression with the particular risk of neutropenic sepsis is also seen.

Bone marrow transplantation carries the added risks of graft versus host disease and prolonged immunosuppression.

Total body irradiation during marrow transplantation may cause pneumonitis.

CNS prophylaxis in young children may have effects on later intellectual development. Attempts are constantly being made to minimize this effect by reducing the dose and field of CNS irradiation.

Testicular irradiation will result in sterility but not impotence.

Prognosis

The prognosis for childhood ALL is for around 70 per cent of children to be long-term survivors cured of their disease. In adults only about half this number will survive free from relapse 3 years after diagnosis. Bone marrow transplantation in this group may improve on these figures.

Acute myeloid leukaemia (AML)

Epidemiology

AML has an incidence of around 4 in 100 000 in the UK, affecting males and females in approximately equal proportions. It is most common in young children under the age of 4 years and in adults over 40 years.

Aetiology

Radiation exposure

Populations exposed after nuclear explosions in Hiroshima and Nagasaki, and after therapeutic or diagnostic use of radiation when it is a rare but recognized event.

Alkylating agents

This includes in particular drugs such as chlorambucil.

The vast majority of cases of AML (over 90 per cent) have no clear association with environmental agents and appear to arise *de novo*.

Pathology

AML encompasses a much broader pathological spectrum of disease than ALL. The characteristics of the myeloblast are positive staining with Sudan black and peroxidase stains. Eight subtypes based on morphological and cytochemical differences are now recognized; their features are outlined in Table 17.3.

Table 17.3   Subtypes of AML

AML subtype	Cell type
M0	Undifferentiated myeloblastic
M1	Undifferentiated myeloblastic without maturation
M2	Differentiated myeloblastic
M3	Promyelocytic
M4	Myelomonocytic
M5	Monoblastic
M6	Erythroleukaemia
M7	Megakaryoblastic

The common forms of AML are M1 and M2. Clinically all these forms of AML behave in a similar fashion.

Around half of all patients with AML will have chromosomal abnormalities. Recognized changes include trisomy of chromosome 8, deletions affecting chromosome 5 or 7 and abnormalities of chromosome 11, all of which are poor prognostic features.

Natural history

There is progressive infiltration of the bone marrow with subsequent bone marrow failure.

Testicular and CNS involvement is relatively rare. CNS involvement is most common in monoblastic AML.

Extramedullary involvement is more common than with ALL with infiltration of liver and spleen in over 50 per cent and characteristic skin and gum infiltration in myelomonocytic and monoblastic leukaemias.

Symptoms

Symptoms include bone marrow failure causing, fatigue, recurrent infections and haemorrhage.

There is also associated fever, sweats and weight loss.

Scattered bone pains may also occur.

Signs

- Signs of anaemia, bruising, purpura and recurrent infection may be present.
- Hepatosplenomegaly is common.
- Lymphadenopathy is less common than with ALL.
- Gum hypertrophy with associated gum bleeding may be apparent particularly in myelomonocytic and monoblastic forms of AML.

Differential diagnosis

Other forms of acute leukaemia and non-Hodgkin's lymphoma together with aplastic anaemia and myelofibrosis should be considered.

Investigations

A full blood count will show pancytopenia with the presence of primitive blast cells on examining the blood film.

Routine biochemistry may show abnormalities in liver function due to infiltration and chest X-ray may show signs of infection or more rarely leukaemic infiltration.

There may be coagulation abnormalities particularly with promyelocytic leukaemia which is associated with disseminated intravascular coagulation.

The diagnosis will be confirmed on examination of the bone marrow and the subtype of AML determined by specific stains.

Treatment

Induction

This consists of chemotherapy in the form of daunorubicin, cytosine arabinoside and thioguanine or etoposide (DAT). This will produce complete regression in up to 85 per cent of patients on first exposure to these agents.

Consolidation

Consolidation therapy in AML is less standardized than for ALL and may either consist of further courses of DAT or alternative chemotherapy such as high dose cytosine arabinoside. Patients with CNS disease will also require cranial irradiation and intrathecal methotrexate but prophylactic CNS treatment is not generally recommended in contrast to ALL.

Maintenance

Maintenance therapy has not been shown to have great value in AML and chemotherapy is not usually continued beyond 6 months after achieving initial remission.

Bone marrow transplantation

This has a role in the management of AML and is considered in some centres as the consolidation treatment of choice for young adults using either an allograft or autograft. It may also be considered in selected patients who relapse after primary treatment particularly those who achieve a second remission with standard chemotherapy.

Tumour-related complications

These include in particular the effects of pancytopenia including anaemia, susceptibility to infection and haemorrhage.

Treatment-related complications

Chemotherapy may be associated with further bone marrow depression and in particular the risk of neutropenic sepsis. Bone marrow transplant has its own specific risks of infection, graft versus host disease and radiation induced pneumonitis.

Prognosis

The prognosis for AML is not as good as for ALL but has improved considerably in recent years with the use of bone marrow transplantation. Overall around 40 per cent of all patients are cured of AML. Cure rates of around 50 per cent are to be expected in those undergoing transplantation in first remission and 25 per cent for those who are transplanted in second remission. Poor prognostic features at presentation include a high white count greater than 100 x 10⁹/l and disseminated intravascular coagulation associated with M3. The outlook is worse for older patients (over 40 years) who have a lower rate of initial remission and are less able to tolerate intensive chemotherapy regimes or bone marrow transplantation.

Chronic leukaemia

Epidemiology

Chronic leukaemias are malignancies of cells which have differentiated beyond the blast stage. They do not, however, despite their name, necessarily have a more protracted natural history and the prognosis for chronic leukaemia is overall no better than for acute leukaemia.

Chronic granulocytic leukaemia (CGL)

CGL typically affects adults between the ages of 30 and 60 years. Its annual incidence in the UK is around 0.8 in 100 000 and it affects men and women equally.

Aetiology

There are no recognized environmental agents.

Philadelphia chromosome is present in around 80 per cent of patients formed by a translocation from chromosome 22 to chromosome 9 or less frequently another chromosome. Additional chromosomal abnormalities frequently develop in the acute phase of CGL (the blast crisis).

Pathology

CGL represents neoplastic proliferation of differentiated granulocytes and is characterized by an excess of metamyelocytes and myelocytes in the peripheral blood. Promyelocytes and myeloblasts may also be present and often there is an excess of basophils and eosinophils.

Natural history

An initial indolent period gives way to a fulminating blast crisis indistinguishable from an acute leukaemia but in general is less responsive to treatment.

Blast crisis is usually myeloblastic in type although lymphoblastic crises may occur. Occasionally the blast crisis may be the first clinical manifestation of the disease when it can be distinguished from a *de novo* acute leukaemia by the presence of Philadelphia chromosome.

Symptoms

Chronic phase CGL may present with symptoms of anaemia or thrombocytopenia due to bone marrow failure.

Abdominal distension and discomfort may occur due to splenic enlargement which may be massive.

Bone pain may also be present.

General features of an active leukaemic process such as fevers and weight loss may occur and patients may also complain of itching.

The very high white count may result in hyperviscosity of the blood causing confusion and headaches.

Priapism is a further rare complication.

Signs

- Clinical signs of anaemia and purpura may be present.
- Massive splenomegaly.
- Hepatomegaly.
- Lymphadenopathy may be present but is usually not prominent.

Differential diagnosis

Myelofibrosis may also present with a large spleen and pancytopenia.

In the acute phase differentiation between *de novo* acute leukaemia and blast crisis of CGL may be difficult unless the preceding history is known but can be resolved by the finding of Philadelphia chromosome.

Investigations

The peripheral blood usually has a characteristic picture with a very high white blood cell count of between 100 and 1000 x 10^9/l of which the majority will be metamyelocytes with other granulocyte precursors. This is usually associated with a mild thrombocytopenia and anaemia.

Bone marrow examination should also be performed which will show a hypercellular picture with an excess of granulocyte precursors. Areas of myelosclerosis may also be seen. Philadelphia chromosome may be demonstrated in myeloid, erythroid and megakaryocytic cell lines.

Abdominal ultrasound may be performed to confirm the extent of hepatomegaly and splenomegaly.

Other characteristic abnormalities are a low leucocyte alkaline phosphatase and raised serum B12 and B12 binding proteins.

Blast crisis is characterized by the appearance of more primitive blast cells and on bone marrow these will comprise over 50 per cent of the myeloid population.

Treatment

Chronic phase

Initial treatment is aimed at reducing the peripheral blood white cell count to under $15 \times 10^9/l$ and to alleviate symptoms of splenomegaly.

Chemotherapy using busulphan taken as a daily oral dose of 4 mg may be used until the white cell count reaches satisfactory levels. This is usually paralleled by a reduction in spleen size and a return to normal of other markers of CGL such as leucocyte alkaline phosphatase and B12 binding proteins.

Low dose maintenance oral busulphan may be continued or intermittent courses given to maintain the white cell count within normal limits.

Ultimately many patients become resistant to busulphan at which time alternative agents may be introduced such as hydroxyurea, 6-mercaptopurine, chlorambucil or cyclophosphamide. There is also interest in the use of interferon to maintain patients in the chronic phase in remission.

Splenic irradiation may be useful in the palliation of local symptoms from a large spleen and the effects of hypersplenism in disease refractory to chemotherapy.

Leucophoresis will achieve rapid reduction of very high white cell counts. The patient's blood is passed through a cell separator being returned through a continuous flow into a second intravenous cannula. This results on average in a 35 per cent reduction in white cell count with each procedure, and also has the advantage of providing large numbers of redundant granulocytes which can be used for therapeutic transfusion in other patients. However, no effect on the natural history of the CGL process is achieved by regular leucophoresis and it is therefore generally used only when hyperviscosity is a predominant feature.

The role of more intensive chemotherapy in the chronic phase of CGL is still under evaluation but there are encouraging reports of prolonged remissions after allogeneic bone marrow transplant.

Acute phase

The treatment of the blast crisis is essentially that of the acute leukaemia into which the CGL transforms. In around 70 per cent this will be an acute myeloid leukaemia, around 5 per cent may have a mixed picture and the remaining 25 per cent will manifest ALL. As with *de novo* acute leukaemia an ALL blast crisis has a better prognosis with around 40 per cent of patients reverting to a chronic phase with simple induction therapy such as vincristine and prednisolone. Bone marrow transplantation may be of value in those patients achieving remission from their acute phase.

Tumour-related complications

There may be bone marrow failure resulting in anaemia, reduced resistance to infection and a bleeding tendency due to thrombocytopenia. This may be exacerbated by the effects of gross splenomegaly causing the phenomenon of hypersplenism with pooling of blood within the large spleen.

Massive splenomegaly may also cause local pain and may impair gastric emptying. Local areas of infarction may occur within the spleen causing acute pain.

Large numbers of white cells in the circulation may cause hyper-viscosity with headache, confusion, visual disturbance and priapism.

Treatment-related complications

Busulphan is associated with a rare Addisonian-like syndrome in which there is pigmentation, hyponatraemia and weakness. Other features which are occasionally seen include pulmonary fibrosis, amenorrhoea, gynaecomastia and testicular atrophy.

Bone marrow depression may occur due to chemotherapy resulting in further anaemia, infection and bleeding.

Splenic irradiation or surgical splenectomy may be hazardous because of thrombocytopenia and a subsequent predisposition to infection, particularly pneumococcal pneumonia.

Rapid lysis of large populations of leukaemic cells may result in hyperuricaemia although florid gout is rare as is tumour lysis syndrome. This is prevented by the use of allopurinol with chemotherapy and ensuring adequate fluid input.

Prognosis

The median survival of patients with CGL is around 4 years with death usually occurring in the acute blast crisis. This, however, masks the fact that some patients may live for many years in the chronic phase and an increasing number of patients are entering durable remissions in the acute phase with high dose treatment and bone marrow transplantation.

Chronic lymphocytic leukaemia (CLL)

CLL represents the end of the leukaemic spectrum where the classification merges with that of non-Hodgkin's lymphoma. CLL is a neoplastic proliferation of the same cell type as lymphocytic lymphoma, the differentiating feature being the extent of bone marrow infiltration.

Epidemiology

CLL affects a somewhat older age group than CGL, with patients predominantly over 60 years. Males and females are affected in approximately equal proportions.

Aetiology

No specific aetiological factors for the common form of CLL seen in Europe and America have been recognized.

The rarer T-cell variant may be associated with HTLV1 infection, as found in Japan and the Caribbean.

Around half of all patients with CLL have demonstrable chromosomal abnormalities. The most common of these is trisomy of chromosome 12 with chromosome 14 being abnormal in other patients.

Pathology

The cell of origin for CLL is in most cases a B lymphocyte although in 5 per cent there may be markers of T-cell origin. The B-cell type will demonstrate surface immunoglobulin which may be either kappa or lambda. The characteristic finding in the peripheral blood is of large numbers of mature lymphocytes with a total lymphocyte count of over 5000 x 10⁹/l being required to confirm the diagnosis. This is associated with bone marrow infiltration by immature lymphocytes which should account for more than 30 per cent of the total marrow. Three patterns of marrow involvement have been described: interstitial, nodular or diffuse. As with non-Hodgkin's lymphomas diffuse appearance is associated with a worse prognosis than the more focal forms.

Natural history

The natural history spans many years. Ultimately death may occur due to bone marrow failure or to transformation into a high grade lymphoma.

Symptoms

- May be asymptomatic for some time.
- Painless lymphadenopathy.
- Symptoms of anaemia.
- Recurrent infections may also occur.
- Fever, sweats and weight loss are the common systemic manifestations.

Signs

- Peripheral lymphadenopathy.
- Splenomegaly
- Hepatomegaly may also occur but is usually only mild.

Investigations

A full blood count will reveal anaemia, thrombocytopenia and a high total white cell count which on examination of the blood film is predominantly small, round, lymphocytes.

Bone marrow examination will confirm the diagnosis with the finding of excess lymphoid cells, at least 30 per cent of which will be immature forms.

Hypogammaglobulinaemia is a common association.

Haemolytic anaemia may be associated with CLL with elevated conjugated bilirubin and a positive Coomb's test.

Lymph node biopsy may be performed which will show infiltration of involved nodes with well-differentiated lymphocytes, usually in a diffuse pattern.

In HTLV-associated CLL hypercalcaemia and hyponatremia are characteristic features.

Differential diagnosis

Non-Hodgkin's lymphoma should be considered, particularly the diffuse small cell types.

Treatment

Because CLL has a long indolent course, in most patients treatment is only considered when symptomatic. There is usually a good response to gentle oral chemotherapy using chlorambucil or cyclophosphamide which can often be discontinued after several months until either the white count rises excessively or other local symptoms from enlarged nodes or splenomegaly arise. Steroids may also be used and are of value when the disease becomes refractory to alkylating agents but there is no evidence that adding them to chlorambucil or cyclophosphamide in the early management of the disease is of value. Other combinations have also included vincristine or vinblastine but again no significant advantage over single agent therapy has emerged.

Low dose irradiation will result in rapid shrinkage of enlarged node masses or splenomegaly. Doses as low as 20 or 30 Gy over 2 to 3 weeks are usually sufficient and associated with little or no morbidity.

There is no evidence that high dose intensive treatment produces better results than more gentle therapy and bone marrow transplantation has no established role in CLL.

Tumour-related complications

The associated hypogammaglobulinaemia results in a high incidence of infections.

There may be chronic anaemia which can have a haemolytic component requiring regular transfusions. Thrombocytopenia may also persist.

The rare HTLV-related CLL may be associated with hypercalcaemia.

Treatment-related complications

Oral alkylating agents are usually relatively trouble free provided careful attention is paid to the blood count and treatment stopped when there are signs of significant bone marrow depression.

With a large tumour burden there is always the possibility of provoking hyperuricaemia due to cell lysis on initiation of chemotherapy. This should be prevented by administration of allopurinol and ensuring adequate fluid intake.

Prognosis

While remissions are usually readily achieved in CLL cures are rare. Many patients will live with their disease for several years, the median survival being around 8 years.

The HTLV-associated T-cell form of CLL is a far more aggressive disease, however, and patients may succumb within a few months.

Rare forms of leukaemia

Prolymphocytic leukaemia

This is related to CLL, presenting in elderly men with splenomegaly and very high white cell counts. The cells are larger than the mature lymphocytes seen in CLL and the disease has a more aggressive course.

Hairy cell leukaemia

This is a chronic leukaemia occurring in the middle aged and is more frequent in men than women. It is rare accounting for around 2 per cent of all cases of adult leukaemia. Typically it presents with massive splenomegaly and pancytopenia. The characteristic finding is of 'hairy cells' in the peripheral blood and bone marrow. These are B lymphocytes with cytoplasmic projections giving them a 'hairy' appearance under the microscope.

Hairy cell leukaemia usually has a long indolent course. It responds to treatment with interferon with which it may remain in remission for many years before it becomes resistant and bone marrow failure develops.

Multiple myeloma

Epidemiology

The incidence of multiple myeloma in the UK in men is around 45 per million with approximately 2000 cases diagnosed each year. Men and women are affected in equal proportions. There has been an apparent increase in incidence over the past 30 years from only 5 per million in 1960 which probably reflects improved diagnostic abilities rather than a true increase in the prevalence of the disease.

Aetiology

There are no recognized aetiological agents for multiple myeloma. It has been suggested that the origin of the paraprotein production may be as a host antibody response to a foreign protein but no consistent antigen has been identified.

Pathology

Multiple myeloma is one of a spectrum of plasma cell neoplasms which range from benign monoclonal gammopathy through solitary plasmacytoma to multiple myeloma. All these conditions are characterized by a neoplastic proliferation of B cells producing a characteristic paraprotein. Transformation within this group of conditions is well recognized with around 20 per cent of benign monoclonal gammopathies and 70 per cent of apparent solitary plasmacytomas eventually developing multiple myeloma.

Natural History

Once established myeloma affects the bone marrow, bones and kidneys. Bone invasion is facilitated by release of chemicals which act as osteoclast activating factors including interleukins (in particular IL1 and IL6), tumour necrosis factor (TNF) and macrophage colony stimulating factor (M-CSF).

Renal damage occurs due to deposition of paraprotein and amyloid formation, hypercalcaemia and hyperuricaemia.

Symptoms

Symptoms of multiple myeloma typically present in three ways:

1. Bone marrow infiltration causing anaemia; thrombocytopenia is usually not prominent but more commonly there may be a bleeding disorder due to the effects of macroglobulinaemia.
2. Bone destruction resulting in local pain, pathological fracture or neurological complications such as nerve root or spinal cord compression – bone pain is present in two-thirds of patients presenting with myeloma.
3. Metabolic and biochemical disturbance including:

   • High levels of paraprotein causing hyperviscosity, resulting in confusion and headache.
   • Renal failure which is present in around one-third of patients as defined by a raised blood urea which may cause nausea, vomiting, malaise, fluid retention or itching.
   • Hypercalcaemia which is present in around one-third of patients who present with myeloma resulting in thirst, polyuria, dyspepsia, nausea, vomiting, constipation or confusion.

Signs

Clinical signs of myeloma may be few. Patients may be clinically anaemic and bone lesions may present as locally tender or even swollen areas. There may be rib or spinal tenderness.

Patients presenting with pathological fracture will have obvious signs of swelling, tenderness and deformity.

Cord compression may present with weakness of the lower limbs, sphincter disturbance and neurological signs of an upper motor neurone lesion. In contrast cauda equina compression from disease in the lumbosacral spine will result in lower motor neurone weakness.

Hyperviscosity causes confusion.

Papilloedema and retinal haemorrhage are also described.

Differential diagnosis

There are few conditions outside the spectrum of plasma cell neoplasms which will mimic myeloma.

Other causes of bone metastases including primary tumours of the breast, lung, thyroid and prostate should be considered.

In practice the major difficulty is in patients who present with a solitary plasma cell lesion who may have a true solitary plasmacytoma but of whom 70 per cent will eventually manifest the characteristic features of widespread multiple myeloma.

Investigations

A full blood count may show anaemia and the ESR will be raised. The blood film may have rouleaux formation.

Biochemical tests will show a raised total protein and there may be hypercalcaemia, renal failure with raised urea and creatinine and hyperuricaemia.

Protein electrophoresis will demonstrate the characteristic M band containing the paraprotein which may also be quantitatively measured. This will be an IgG in around 50 per cent of patients, IgA in 20 per cent, IgM in 10 per cent and light chain only in 10 per cent. Other rare types of paraprotein include IgD (2 per cent) and heavy chain fragments (1 per cent). In 1 per cent of patients there may be two different M proteins and in 1 per cent the paraprotein may be absent.

The serum β microglobulin is also raised in many patients and is an important marker of disease both for prognosis and for monitoring treatment.

There may be proteinuria and on electrophoresis Bence–Jones protein.

Bone marrow examination will show infiltration with plasma cells; infiltration with more than 10 per cent plasma cells is diagnostic.

An X-ray skeletal survey may show lytic bone lesions, many of which are asymptomatic. Typical appearances are shown on the skull X-ray in Figure 17.1. Because the bone metastases of myeloma are usually predominantly lytic with little osteoblastic reaction they often do not show on isotope bone scan or may be seen as cold areas rather than hot spots.

Fig. 17.1   Lateral skull X-ray showing multiple lytic bone deposits of myeloma.

Other investigations may be considered where indicated, including plasma viscosity, plasma volume, and rectal biopsy for amyloid.

Staging

A number of criteria for the diagnosis of myeloma have been defined. These are shown in Table 17.4

Staging of myeloma is based on recognized prognostic factors which include haemoglobin, blood urea, serum calcium, extent of bone lesions and level of paraprotein. The usual classification applied in the UK is the Durie–Salmon staging system as shown below.

Table 17.4   Criteria for diagnosis of myeloma

1. Presence of a monoclonal 'M' protein in serum or urine
2. Bone lesions due to a plasma cell infiltrate
3. Marrow plasma cells accounting for > 10% of marrow infiltrate.
4. Associated features: anaemia
                        hypercalcaemia
                        renal failure

Diagnosis is confirmed on demonstration of any two of 1 to 3.

Durie–Salmon staging for multiple myeloma
Stage 1 Hb > 10 g/dl

- Calcium normal.
- Normal bone skeletal survey (or solitary plasmacytoma).
- Low serum and urine paraprotein (serum IgG < 6 g/dl; IgA < 3g/dl; urine < 4g/24 h).

Stage 2 Neither stage 1 nor stage 3.

Stage 3 Hb < 8.5 g/dl

- Calcium > 12 mg/dl.
- Multiple lytic bone lesions.
- High paraprotein levels (serum IgG > 7 g/dl; IgA > 5 g/dl; urine > 12 g/24 h).

There is a further subclassification into A (normal renal function) or B (raised serum creatinine)

It is proposed that the staging correlates with plasma cell mass increasing from $< 0.6 \times 10^{12}/m^2$ for stage 1 to $> 1.2 \times 10^{12}/m^2$ for stage 3.

Serum β_2 microglobulin is a further important prognostic indicator.

Treatment

There is a small group of patients with indolent myeloma manifest by a few asymptomatic bone lesions or mild anaemia who require no specific treatment and will be managed by transfusion when appropriate and occasional monitoring of the serum paraprotein and β_2 microglobulin.

Solitary lesions (true plasmacytomas) are usually treated with local radiotherapy alone.

The remainder of patients will require treatment with chemotherapy and where indicated radiotherapy to sites of painful bone lesions.

Chemotherapy for myeloma

There are four main approaches to the drug treatment of myeloma.

Melphelan

To be given as an intermittent oral regime for 5 to 7 days every month. Attempts have been made to increase the efficacy of oral melphelan by adding steroids or vincristine but there is no evidence that this is of any value. Weekly cyclophosphamide injections are sometimes used as an alternative with equivalent results.

Combination chemotherapy

It has recently been shown that a four drug combination therapy is superior to melphelan alone in some patients. The current combination evaluated by the Medical Research Council in the UK is ABCM which comprises adriamycin, BCNU, cyclophosphamide and melphelan.

Steroid-based regimes

It has been shown that continuous infusions of steroids such as dexamethasone are active in myeloma. The addition of other drugs may improve the results of this slightly as in the VAD schedule (vincristine, adriamycin and dexamethasone).

High dose chemotherapy

This is perhaps the single most effective modality for initial treatment, although long-term overall survival may be little better. High dose melphelan has been used in this context with bone marrow autograft following the high dose chemotherapy.

The choice of treatment for an individual patient will depend on both the nature of the disease in that patient and their age and general health. For stage 1 myeloma melphelan alone or in a younger patient ABCM or VAD may be chosen. For stage 3 myeloma high dose therapy should be considered for young patients (< 50 years). For older patients high dose therapy has considerable morbidity and mortality from the procedure and combination therapy with ABCM or VAD will be more appropriate.

Supportive treatment

Alongside chemotherapy management of the complications of myeloma will have a considerable impact on both the quality of life and the survival of the patient.

Anaemia will require blood transfusion.

Infections will require prompt treatment with appropriate antibiotics.

Hypercalcaemia will require active hydration, diuresis and the use of diphophonates. There is some evidence that the prophylactic use of diphophonates such as APD or clodronate may be of value.

Renal failure will require management of fluid balance and in severe cases dialysis may be justified.

Pathological fracture will require internal fixation followed by local radiotherapy.

Active rehabilitation is also important as immobility is a further adverse prognostic factor.

Tumour-related complications

These have been covered in the above discussion on supportive treatment in myeloma.

Treatment-related complications

Chemotherapy will cause bone marrow depression and the blood count must be carefully monitored with aggressive treatment of neutropenic infections. This is particularly the case when high dose therapy is given where there will be a period of 2 to 3 weeks when the patient is pancytopenic.

Steroid infusions may cause Cushingoid symptoms and, particularly in the elderly, fluid retention causing cardiac failure.

Prognosis

The median survival for patients with stage 1 disease is around 4 years falling to only 2 years for stage 3. Those with solitary plasmacytoma in a site other than bone, usually in the head and neck region, have the best prognosis. Poor renal failure and a high β_2 microglobulin are associated with a poor prognosis with survival of less than 1 year.

18

Paediatric cancer

Malignant tumours are rare in children with an incidence of around 100 per million children per year. Despite this, however, they are the most common cause of death in the age groups of up to 14 years. The greatest incidence is under the age of 5 years when around half of all paediatric cancers are diagnosed.

Tumours in children differ from those in adults with relatively more leukaemias and lymphomas and fewer solid epithelial cancers. The general distribution is shown in Table 18.1.

Table 18.1 Frequency and type of common paediatric cancers

Tumour	Incidence
Leukaemia	30%
CNS tumours	20%
Bone and soft tissue	15%
Lymphoma	10%
Neuroblastoma	7%
Nephroblastoma (Wilm's)	7%
Others	11%

Overall the outlook for paediatric malignancy is far better than for adults, with a cure rate of over 50 per cent. Because of the high cure rate there is now increasing emphasis on the long-term effects of treatment, in particular the influence of chemotherapy and radiotherapy on growth and both physical and intellectual development.

Leukaemias in childhood are predominantly acute lymphoblastic or less frequently acute myeloblastic leukaemias. Chronic leukaemia, while recognized, is extremely rare. Details of these conditions have been covered in Chapter 17.

CNS tumours

Around 70 per cent of childhood CNS tumours are astrocytomas, predominantly low grade, the management of which has been covered in Chapter 17.

Of the remainder, the most common is medulloblastoma which accounts for 15–20 per cent of the total.

Medulloblastoma

Epidemiology

Medulloblastomas are more common under 5 years than over 5 years and occur in twice as many boys as girls.

Aetiology

There are no recognized aetiological factors in the development of this tumour other than the small proportion which develop within the context of Gorlin's syndrome.

Pathology

Typically medulloblastoma is a tumour of the posterior fossa arising within the cerebellum. Obstruction of the fourth ventricle or aqueduct may result in secondary hydrocephalus. A characteristic feature of this tumour is its propensity to seeding throughout the neuroaxis so that meningeal deposits may be found at any site both within the skull and down the spinal cord. Blood-borne metastases have been described, particularly in bone, but these are rare.

Microscopically the cells are derived from precursors of neuronal tissue and have a characteristic appearance likened to short carrots, forming circles or rosettes.

Symptoms

In children CNS tumours may have an insidious onset with irritability and failure to achieve appropriate milestones.

Children or their parents may complain of specific difficulties with walking or headache.

Spinal disease may cause nerve root pains and arm or leg weakness.

Signs

Posterior fossa tumours may cause specific signs of cerebellar dysfunction with incoordination, ataxic gait and scanning dysarthria. There may also be lower cranial nerve signs.

Spinal involvement will cause weakness of limbs and sensory changes, particularly the development of nerve root pains.

Hydrocephalus, causing raised intracranial pressure, may in the young child result in bulging of the fontanelle and increased head circumference.

Differential diagnosis

Other tumours of the posterior fossa should be considered of which the most common is a low grade astrocytoma. Unlike adults metastases in the posterior fossa are rare in children.

Investigations

Routine tests such as a full blood count and biochemical screen are usually unremarkable as is routine radiology including a skull X-ray.

The tumour will be seen on CT scan which should be enhanced with intravenous contrast. CT will also demonstrate any degree of hydrocephalus.

MRI is often superior to CT in imaging the posterior fossa and should be used where available. This is shown in Chapter 2, Figure 2.1.

Some form of spinal imaging is essential to complete the staging process. In the past this has required a myelogram but this can now be replaced by MRI scan.

Staging

There is no TNM staging for medulloblastoma, although various other staging systems have been proposed. Essentially patients can be divided by certain prognostic factors into two groups, poor prognosis features being brain stem or supratentorial involvement, age less than 18 months and spinal or distant metastases.

Treatment

Initial treatment following the diagnosis of a posterior fossa tumour will be surgery. Surgery has three roles in the management of this tumour:

1. To confirm the histological diagnosis from resected tissue.
2. To remove all visible tumour if technically possible.
3. To relieve hydrocephalus if present by the insertion of a ventri-culoperitoneal shunt.

Following surgery post-operative radiotherapy will be given. This involves treatment of the whole craniospinal axis, i.e. the whole brain and spinal column down to the level of S2 where the thecal sac terminates.

There may also be some benefit from chemotherapy for high risk patients, i.e. those with brain stem involvement, incomplete surgical removal, supratentorial tumour or spinal tumour.

Tumour-related complications

Obstructive hydrocephalus may occur.

There may be permanent neurological deficits, in particular incoordina-tion and ataxia. Spinal disease may result in permanent limb weakness.

Treatment-related complications

Ventriculoperitoneal shunts may become infected or block requiring surgical revision.

Craniospinal irradiation may cause significant bone marrow depression, particularly in those patients receiving chemotherapy. Late effects of this treatment include impaired growth, particularly of spinal growth resulting in a disproportionate reduction in sitting height compared to standing height. The ovaries are usually included in the sacral radiation field resulting in sterility in young girls.

Pituitary irradiation within the whole brain volume may result in varying degrees of hypopituitarism requiring appropriate replacement therapy.

Late results of whole brain irradiation may result in some blunting of intellectual development and failure to reach the full potential which may have been predicted pre-treatment. Despite this many patients achieve good results and function normally within society.

Prognosis

The overall long-term cure rate is 40–50 per cent.

Rare tumours

Ependymomas

These account for around 8 per cent of childhood brain tumours. When occurring in the posterior fossa they behave in a very similar fashion to medulloblastomas and the principles of treatment are the same. Cure rates are also similar.

Bone and soft tissue

The common bone tumours in children are osteosarcoma and Ewing's sarcoma, both of which are discussed in Chapter 15.

The common soft tissue tumour to occur in children is the embryonal rhabdomyosarcoma. This differs significantly from the alveolar and pleomorphic forms of rhabdomyosarcoma found in adults.

Rhabdomyosarcoma (embryonal type)

Epidemiology

These tumours are usually seen in the first 5 years of life and have an overall incidence of 3 per million children under 15 years of age. They may arise in any site, the most common being the head and neck region and the genitourinary tract.

Aetiology

There are no known aetiological factors.

Pathology

Approximately one-third arise in the head and neck region, one-third in the genitourinary tract and a quarter in the soft tissues of the trunk or extremities. The orbit is also a relatively frequent site accounting for 10 per cent of the total.

Macroscopically they appear as pink fleshy masses and proliferative forms may be likened to bunches of grapes ('sarcoma botryoides').

Microscopically they are embryonal cells which are rich in glycogen and within which myofibrils can be demonstrated.

The natural history of this form of rhabdomyosarcoma is for rapid local growth with infiltration along tissue planes and early blood-borne metastases. Around 1 in 5 will have bone marrow infiltration at presentation. Lymph node spread may also occur, particularly in those tumours arising in the genitourinary tract and limbs.

Symptoms

Presenting symptoms depend on site of origin. Many arise as rapidly enlarging but painless masses. Other local symptoms may be present including nasal obstruction and epistaxis from the nasopharynx, haematuria from the urinary tract, vaginal bleeding from the vagina or uterus and visual disturbances from the orbit.

Signs

Clinical signs will go along with the presenting symptoms. There may be an obvious mass visible. Vaginal tumours may present with a fleshy mass of 'botryoid' tumour at the introitus.

Differential diagnosis

In childhood there are few other tumours which are likely to arise in similar sites to rhabdomyosarcoma. Other causes of presenting symptoms such as epistaxis or haematuria in the absence of an obvious mass will be sought.

Investigations

Routine tests such as full blood count and biochemistry may well be normal.

Chest X-ray may demonstrate lung metastases.

CT scan of the affected site will be valuable in delineating the extent of local tumour most accurately.

Bone marrow examination should be performed in view of the high incidence of marrow involvement and skeletal X-ray survey or isotope bone scan should also be performed.

A full examination of the affected site under anaesthetic with biopsy of the tumour is essential to confirm the diagnosis.

Staging

TNM staging is used and is based on post surgical status:

T1 – Tumour limited to site of origin with microscopic margins of excision clear.
T2 – Tumour extending beyond site of origin but complete microscopic clearance of tumour.
T3 – Tumour extending beyond site of origin with incomplete excision.
N0 – Regional nodes negative
N1 – Regional nodes involved
M0 – No metastases.
M1 – Distant metastases.

Treatment

Radical

Chemotherapy

Given to all cases using VAC (vincristine, actinomycin and cyclophosphamide). One or two courses are given followed by definitive surgery or radiotherapy and then chemotherapy is continued for a period of up to 1 year.

Local treatment will be either:

Surgery

This is the treatment of choice in the absence of advanced distant metastases. For urogenital, truncal and limb rhabdomyosarcoma wide resection is usually performed.

or

Radiotherapy

Used for inoperable tumours such as orbit and nasopharynx, delivering doses of around 50 Gy in 5 weeks.

Palliative

For disseminated disease a course of palliative chemotherapy or radiotherapy may be valuable in minimizing symptoms.

Tumour-related complications

These will depend on the site. Urogenital tumours may permanently affect renal, urinary and reproductive function and orbital tumours may affect sight.

Treatment-related complications

Chemotherapy using VAC may cause nausea, vomiting and alopecia during the period of administration. In the longer term peripheral neuropathy from vincristine can persist.

Radical surgery may have late sequelae depending on the type of procedure. There are obvious effects of cystectomy or hysterectomy for urogenital tumours.

Radical radiotherapy may have late sequelae also, in particular growth impairment in the treated area. In a young child this can result in quite marked disfigurement if significant asymmetry develops, as may be the case following, for example, orbit irradiation.

Prognosis

The overall prognosis for embryonal rhabdomyosarcoma which is confined to the site of origin is good with cure rates of around 80 per cent. Once metastatic the outlook is poor with less than 20 per cent surviving.

Site is an important predictor of cure. The best prognoses are associated with tumours of the orbit, bladder, paratesticular region and vagina. Poor prognosis sites are parameningeal, prostate and perineum.

Lymphoma

Both Hodgkin's disease and non-Hodgkin's lymphoma may occur in children. While they obey the general rules discussed in the Chapter 16 there are certain features of paediatric lymphomas which should be considered.

Non-Hodgkin's lymphoma

NHL in children is usually high grade nodal disease with a particular propensity for diffuse lymphoblastic or undifferentiated tumours and also T-cell lymphomas associated with a mediastinal mass. Low grade NHL is rare in children.

Treatment usually involves combination chemotherapy and for extensive high grade disease bone marrow transplant may be considered. Local radiotherapy may also be given in doses of 25–30 Gy.

Hodgkin's disease

Hodgkin's disease is relatively more common in boys than in girls which is in contrast to a more even sex distribution in adults. Lymphocyte-predominant histology is relatively more common and the less favourable lymphocyte-depleted form uncommon.

Treatment is based on the same principles as in adult Hodgkin's disease but with even greater emphasis on minimizing late effects. For this reason chemotherapy is often preferred for relatively early disease avoiding the local growth problems after radiotherapy. Where irradiation is used lower doses of around 30 Gy are given compared to 35–40 Gy in adults.

Neuroblastoma

Epidemiology

Neuroblastoma is a tumour of young children, 50 per cent occurring before the age of 2 years. It has an annual incidence of 8 per million and is slightly more common in boys than in girls. There is some geographical variation, being rare in Africa compared to Europe and America.

Aetiology

There is an association with Von Recklinghausen's disease (multiple neurofibromatosis) and colonic aganglionosis, but most cases have no recognizable causal factor. There is some evidence that it may arise as a congenital anomaly and cases *in utero* have been reported.

Specific chromosome abnormalities have been identified in neuroblastoma including amplification of small chromosome segments and deletions affecting chromosome 1.

Pathology

Two-thirds of neuroblastomas are intra-abdominal tumours of which 60 per cent occur in the adrenal and 40 per cent at other sites related to the sympathetic chain. The remaining third are divided between the chest, pelvis and head and neck region. In a small number of these tumours widespread metastatic disease may be present with no recognizable primary site.

Macroscopically the tumour is usually encapsulated but soft and friable, containing areas of haemorrhage, necrosis, cystic degeneration and calcification.

Microscopically there is a spectrum of appearances depending on the degree of differentiation. Typically it is composed of densely packed, small round cells which may form rosettes. In the more differentiated forms neurofibrils and ganglionic elements and granule-containing chromaffin cells may be seen.

Natural history

Local infiltration of surrounding tissues is seen.

Regional lymph nodes may be involved but the predominant pattern of metastases is by early blood-borne dissemination with around two-thirds of children having widespread disease at presentation, affecting in particular bone and liver. Lung metastases are relatively rare.

Spontaneous maturation and regression may occur. At post-mortem there is a much higher incidence of asymptomatic tumours in patients dying from unrelated conditions than in the general population.

Symptoms

These will depend on the site and age at presentation.

Abdominal tumours which are the most common will present with abdominal discomfort and bowel or urinary obstruction.

In the head and neck a painless mass may be the first manifestation.

There also may be fever, anorexia, malaise and weight loss.

Metastatic disease may cause the first symptoms, particularly bone pain from bone metastases.

Excessive catecholamine production from the tumour cells causes flushing, palpitations, diarrhoea and headache.

Rarely *in utero* it presents with pre-eclampsia in the mother.

Signs

A palpable mass may be apparent.

Intrathoracic tumours may cause venous obstruction with dilated neck veins, plethora and oedema.

Catecholamine secretion may cause hypertension.

There are rare neurological syndromes associated with neuroblastoma, in particular an acute cerebellar disturbance.

Differential diagnosis

A tumour presenting as a palpable mass must be distinguished from other types of tumour. In the abdomen this will include Wilm's tumour and in the neck a lymph node due to lymphoma.

The differential diagnosis of a small round cell tumour in bone includes not only neuroblastoma but also Ewing's sarcoma and lymphoma.

Investigations

Routine blood tests may be unremarkable but extensive bone metastases may cause pancytopenia and there may be obstructive renal impairment.

X-ray of the tumour may demonstrate speckled calcification within it.

CT or MRI is needed for more accurate definition of the tumour.

A bone marrow examination is important because of the high incidence of bone metastases.

Twenty-four hour urine collections will be made to measure catecholamines as vanillylmandelic acid (VMA) and homovanillylmandelic acid (HVA), the ratio of the two having prognostic importance. Other peptides such as vasoactive intestinal peptide (VIP) may also be raised.

Because many of the tumours will contain cells synthesizing catecholamines from their precursors a labelled precursor called meta-iodo-benzyl guanidine (MIBG) may be used as a tracer to be used in scanning when labelled with radioactive iodine. This also has therapeutic uses.

Staging

The Audrey Evans classification is used:

Stage 1   Confined to the site of origin.

Stage 2   Extending beyond site of origin but not crossing midline.

Stage 3   Extending beyond site of origin across midline.

Stage 4   Distant metastases.

Stage 4S Infants (<2 years) with local tumour not crossing midline but with liver, skin or bone marrow metastases.

Treatment

Stages 1 and 2

Local treatment alone is given by radical surgical excision.
Post-operative radiotherapy is given for older children (>1 year) or those with poorly differentiated tumours. Neuroblastoma is very sensitive to irradiation and doses of only 20–30 Gy over 3 to 4 weeks are adequate.

Stages 3 and 4

Chemotherapy using a combination of cyclophosphamide and vincristine with the addition of adriamycin, etoposide or cisplatin is given in those over 1 year of age.

Intensive chemotherapy using high doses of drugs such as melphelan with or without autologous bone marrow transplant may be considered.

Targeted radiation using Iodine[131]-labelled MIBG, which is actively concentrated in cells synthesising catecholamines, is also used.

Palliative treatment

Local radiotherapy for painful bone metastases or large tumour masses may be used.

Stage 4S disease

With little or no treatment spontaneous regression of tumour occurs.

Vincristine or low dose irradiation may be indicated for pressure symptoms due to a large liver or other tumour mass.

Tumour-related complications

Mediastinal, renal or intestinal obstruction may occur, depending on primary site.

Excess catecholamine secretion may cause hypertension and tachycardia with arrhythmias. Diarrhoea may occur if VIP is produced.

Treatment-related complications

Irradiation of the abdomen of a child may cause bowel or renal damage. It is important to design symmetrical fields of irradiation to minimize deformity from growth retardation.

Prognosis

The prognosis for localized neuroblastoma is good with virtually all patients with stage 1 disease and 80 per cent of those with stage 2 cured. Stage 4S also has a good outlook with cure rates approaching 80 per cent. In contrast patients with metastatic disease have a very poor prognosis with less than 10 per cent surviving.

Nephroblastoma (Wilm's tumour)

Epidemiology

Wilm's tumour is a tumour of young children with a peak incidence at 3 years and the majority occurring before the age of 5 years. The annual incidence is 1 in 20 000 children and there is equal distribution between boys and girls.

Aetiology

Wilm's tumour is occasionally familial.

There is an association with certain rare congenital abnormalities including aniridia, hemi-hypertrophy and other abnormalities of the urogenital tract.

A deletion on the short arm of chromosome 11 is thought to be an important event in the development of Wilm's tumour.

Pathology

The tumour arises in the kidney and 5 per cent are bilateral. It may be lobular and is surrounded by a pseudocapsule as it compresses surrounding tissue. There may be areas of haemorrhage, necrosis and cyst formation.

Microscopically there is often considerable variety within the tumour with areas of primitive mesenchymal cells which may show differentiation into fat, muscle or cartilage within which are areas of recognizable embryonal glomerular and renal tubular elements.

Certain microscopic features are of prognostic importance. Sarcomatous, anaplastic or clear cell variants are all associated with a worse prognosis.

Natural history

Local invasion from the renal parenchyma into the renal pelvis and renal vein will occur.

Lymph node involvement is relatively infrequent.

Blood-borne metastases are the usual means of spread beyond the kidney, the most common distant site being the lungs.

Symptoms

Abdominal pain is the most common presenting feature. Haematuria occurs in about 20 per cent and a similar proportion may have unexplained fevers. Other systemic symptoms, however, are unusual.

Pulmonary metastases may cause cough, haemoptysis or dyspnoea.

Signs

The majority have a palpable abdominal mass at presentation which may be entirely asymptomatic.

Hypertension may be present but is relatively unusual.

Differential diagnosis

Abdominal neuroblastoma; usually greater systemic upset and bone metastases rather than lung metastases.

Investigations

A full blood count may show anaemia and urea and electrolytes may be disturbed.

Urinalysis may show both blood and protein in the urine.

Chest X-ray may demonstrate lung metastases.

The primary tumour will be demonstrated on abdominal ultrasound and on IVU. CT scan of the abdomen will give further information about its local extent.

Staging

The largest group investigating Wilm's tumour is the National Wilm's Tumour Study Group in the US and their staging system is commonly reported.

Stage 1 Tumour completely excised and retained within capsule.

Stage 2 Tumour completely excised but extending beyond capsule.

Stage 3 Tumour incompletely excised but no blood-borne metastases.

Stage 4 Blood-borne distant metastases.

Stage 5 Bilateral tumours.

Treatment

Surgery by laparotomy and radical resection of the tumour is performed, which will usually entail a nephroureterectomy and regional node dissection. An important feature of the operation should be mobilisation and careful inspection of the contralateral kidney in view of the significant incidence of bilateral tumours.

Post-operative radiotherapy or chemotherapy are used as follows:

Stage 1 disease is given a short course of weekly vincristine injections.

Stages 2 and 3 disease are given radiotherapy to the renal bed delivering 20–30 Gy in 3 to 4 weeks together with chemotherapy using vincristine and actinomycin D.

Stage 4 disease is treated with more intensive chemotherapy using vincristine, actinomycin D, adriamycin and cyclophosphamide. In patients who respond satisfactorily radiotherapy to the renal bed may also be considered.

Palliative treatment

This may take the form of chemotherapy or local radiotherapy to symptomatic disease. For chemotherapy-resistant lung disease low dose whole lung irradiation may be given delivering 10–12 Gy in 7 or 8 small fractions.

Tumour-related complications

In bilateral tumours preservation of as much renal tissue as possible will be attempted.

Treatment-related complications

Radiotherapy to the renal bed will include the lumbar vertebrae and there will therefore be growth retardation in this area. Because of this it is extremely important that the radiotherapist includes the entire width of the vertebral body to avoid a scoliotic deformity due to differential growth across the vertebral body.

Immediate side effects of chemotherapy may include nausea, vomiting and alopecia. In the longer term vincristine may be associated with a peripheral neuropathy, actinomycin D with liver dysfunction and adriamycin with dose-related cardiomyopathy.

Prognosis

Wilm's tumour is both radio- and chemosensitive and the prognosis for localized disease is therefore very good with 80–90 per cent of patients with stage 1 or 2 disease being cured. Even those presenting with distant metastases (stage 4) have a cure rate of up to 40 per cent.

Other tumours

Histiocytosis X

This is a complex condition arising from a proliferation of histiocytes. Three distinct forms are recognized:

Letterer–Siwe disease

This affects infants and is usually rapidly fatal due to widespread infiltration of liver, spleen, skin and lymph nodes with proliferating histiocytes.

Hand–Schuller–Christian disease

This may occur at any age with a less fulminant course and is once again characterized by widespread infiltration by histiocytes which in this case is characterized by intracellular accumulation of lipid. Bones in particular are affected and patients survive for many years, although most ultimately succumb. It may be treated using drug combinations such as VAC (vincristine, adriamycin or actinomycin D and cyclophosphamide).

Eosinophilic granuloma

The least aggressive form of the disease it is usually localized presenting as solitary lytic bone lesions. Deposits around the pituitary are a recognized cause of diabetes insipidus. They are characterized by accumulations of lipid-filled histiocytes, eosinophils and giant cells. They may regress spontaneously. If symptomatic they respond well to low doses of irradiation.

Retinoblastoma

This is a rare tumour present in around 1 in 20 000 live births. It may follow an autosomal dominant pattern of inheritance although many have no preceding family history. A specific gene translocation has been identified in retinoblastoma with a deletion in the long arm of chromosome 13.

It usually presents in the first 2 years of life with reduced vision, white pupils or strabismus. As the tumour occludes fluid drainage within the eye secondary glaucoma may develop. The diagnosis is confirmed on examination of both eyes under anaesthetic.

Small tumours may be treated by light coagulation using a xenon arc laser or cryotherapy. Larger tumours may be treated with radiotherapy which may be delivered either by placing over the tumour cobalt discs or with external beam treatment where most of the eye has to be included. Enucleation is avoided but may be necessary if the optic nerve is invaded.

Most tumours are cured using this approach with preservation of vision.

Germ cell tumours

Teratomas may present in the first 5 years. The majority are benign but 20 per cent or so will be malignant. The common sites are the ovary and the sacrococcygeal region but they may also be found in the mediastinum, neck, nasopharynx, retroperitoneum or brain.

The management of these tumours is essentially that of germ cell tumours in the adult. Initial treatment will be surgical removal where possible followed by appropriate adjuvant chemotherapy using combinations such as BEP (bleomycin, etoposide and cisplatin). Local radiotherapy may be considered where surgical excision is not feasible, as in the brain. Overall the prognosis, as in adult germ cell tumours, is good.

19

Skin cancer

The skin is the largest organ in the body. Its large surface area and location make it particularly vulnerable to environmental carcinogens. Recent cultural, economic and environmental changes have resulted in many more people being exposed to high levels of ultraviolet radiation. As this is the main risk factor for developing skin cancer, many more cases can be expected in the decades to come.

Squamous cell carcinoma and basal cell carcinoma

Epidemiology

There are 27 000 new cases and 500 deaths (nearly all from squamous cell carcinoma) registered in the UK per annum. Basal cell carcinoma (BCC) is twice as common as squamous cell carcinoma (SCC). The peak incidence is at 60–80 years and it is exceptional in the under 40s in whom a strong aetiological factor can usually be identified, e.g. Gorlin's syndrome, arsenic exposure. There is a slight male predominance and they are more common in caucasians living in a sunny climate, particularly South Africa and Australia, the incidence increasing as one moves closer to the equator. They are only rarely encountered in dark-skinned races.

Aetiology

Ultraviolet radiation is the most important cause accounting for the geographical and racial distribution of skin cancers. They are therefore most frequent on sun-exposed areas of the body.

Previous radiotherapy may lead to skin cancer at the entry or exit site of the radiation. Radiation-induced cancers were a particular problem to the pioneering radiologists who used to calibrate their X-ray machines by exposing their hands to a dose sufficient to cause erythema of the skin.

Tar and soot are rich in aromatic hydrocarbons. SCC of the scrotum was described in 19th century chimney sweeps where soot had become trapped in the rugose skin of the scrotum. Similarly, occupational exposure to tar and bitumen may lead to tumours on the exposed skin and mineral oils were the cause of SCC described in yarn workers where they were used to lubricate the mulespinners. Arsenic is a potent cause of skin cancers and a history of exposure should be sought in patients with multiple BCCs and SCCs. It was once used as a 'tonic' and is found in some pesticides.

SCC has been described arising in chronic varicose (Marjolin's) ulcers, burn scars, cutaneous TB, sinuses from chronic osteomyelitis, and epidermolysis bullosa.

Gorlin's syndrome is a very rare, dominantly inherited syndrome predisposing to multiple BCCs and should be considered in all cases arising under 40 years of age. Palmar pits are characteristic but other features include bifid ribs, a calcified falx cerebris, frontal bossing of the skull and mandibular cysts. Xeroderma pigmentosum is even rarer, recessively inherited, and patients inevitably develop multiple BCCs and SCCs at a very young age.

Chronic immunosuppression by agents such as azothioprine and cyclosporin in organ transplant recipients is associated with an increased incidence of BCC and SCC.

Pathology

The tumours usually arise on sun exposed-skin such as the scalp, nose, ears, periorbital tissues, and dorsum of hand. BCCs are very rare in non-hair bearing skin such as the palms and soles. They are frequently multiple, with changes of solar damage in surrounding skin such as keratoses. An invasive SCC may arise in an area of *in situ* carcinoma such as Bowen's disease. SCCs are usually well circumscribed, appearing as nodules, nodules with some central ulceration (Fig. 19.1) or frank ulcers with raised, everted, nodular edges. BCCs have characteristic telangiectasia and a 'pearly' appearance when nodular (Fig. 19.2). They vary greatly in rate of growth, some persisting unnoticed for many years, others growing rapidly over a period of several months. Large, neglected tumours are accompanied by local tissue destruction and secondary infection. Both BCCs and SCCs may occur concurrently in the same patient.

Microscopically, these tumours are locally invasive, often for some distance beyond their macroscopic margins. The cell of origin of a BCC is uncertain, but thought to be a basal cell of a hair follicle giving rise to small dark staining cells. SCCs arise from keratinocytes, are well differentiated, demonstrate intercellular bridges on electron microscopy and produce keratin. Sometimes the appearances are those of a mixed 'basisquamous' tumour.

Natural history

Both types of tumour are characterized by relentless local infiltration of the surrounding skin and normal tissues lying deep to or adjacent to the skin leading to their eventual destruction.

About 5 per cent of SCCs and less than 1 per cent of BCCs spread to the regional lymph nodes.

Fig. 19.1 A typical squamous cell carcinoma arising on the face. Note the nodular appearance with some central ulceration (Courtesy of Dr. D. Tait).

Fig. 19.2 A basal cell carcinoma with pearly appearance and telangiectasia.

Haematogenous spread is rare for SCCs and virtually unknown for BCCs. Lung and bone are the most common sites of metastatic spread.

Symptoms

The patient may be asymptomatic, the lesion being noticed at a routine medical examination, or the patient may complain of a skin lesion which is causing concern or cosmetic defect. Ulcerating lesions may bleed spontaneously if traumatized and irritation is a common complaint although pain is exceptional.

Signs

Careful inspection under a bright light with a magnifying glass is recommended as it is the most accurate way of defining the macroscopic extent of the tumour which may be much greater than naked eye inspection would suggest. Telangiectasia suggests a BCC. Otherwise, it may be difficult to distinguish a SCC from a BCC by appearance alone. The tumour may be tethered or fixed to underlying tissues depending on the depth of invasion. There may be much destruction of the surrounding tissues and secondary infection of the tumour. Regional lymph nodes should be examined in all cases.

Differential diagnosis

This includes:

1. Keratoacanthoma – this is a benign lesion. It is confused with a SCC and may grow very rapidly to form a large conical lesion with a characteristic central pit filled with keratin. It never spreads beyond the skin and usually resolves spontaneously within several weeks/months.
2. Solar keratosis – this is a benign lesion seen in sun-damaged skin. It is usually a hyperkeratotic plaque with no evidence of nodularity or ulceration or invasion of the adjacent tissues.

Investigations

It is necessary to obtain a tissue diagnosis in all cases prior to treatment.

Skin scraping cytology

This is the least traumatic means of obtaining a sample for analysis. In the hands of a skilled cytopathologist it is a sensitive test and can give a result within hours but equivocal or obviously inconsistent results mean that a biopsy is necessary.

Incisional biopsy

A wedge of tissue is removed taking care to include representative tumour and surrounding normal skin. This is usually performed when the lesion is too extensive to be treated with surgery.

Excisional biopsy

This is best for small lesions that can be easily excised as it provides an accurate histological diagnosis and may be curative if microscopically complete.

Fine needle aspiration of any enlarged regional lymph nodes

This should rarely be required at presentation as palpable lymph-adenopathy is rare.

Radiological investigations

Plain radiographs or a limited CT scan are indicated for very large, deeply invasive tumours to delineate their margins when planning treatment.

Staging

There is no formal staging system in routine clinical use.

Treatment

Both surgery and radiotherapy achieve local control in about 95 per cent of cases. The choice is dependent on the anatomical site, convenience and previous treatment.

Surgery

This is the treatment of choice for:

1. Local recurrences after radiotherapy.
2. Tumours arising in regions which do not tolerate radiotherapy well, e.g. lower third of tibia.
3. Very large tumours involving bone where osteonecrosis is a risk after radiotherapy.
4. Scalp lesions where the patient does not wish to have an area of permanent alopecia.
5. Tumours of the upper eyelid where radiotherapy scarring could cause repeated trauma to the cornea.
6. Young patients in whom the late cutaneous effects of radiotherapy will have longer to become manifest.
7. Patients who can only attend the hospital for a single treatment and in whom the cosmetic outcome is important.

Excision is performed under local anaesthetic, although large lesions requiring a skin graft for reconstruction may be removed under general anaesthetic. Facial lesions are best dealt with by a plastic surgeon to optimize the cosmetic result. Complete macroscopic and micro-scopic excision will be curative for SCC and BCC and so a margin of macroscopically normal skin of up to 10 mm (depending on size of tumour and how well circumscribed it is) should be taken away en bloc. Skin grafting or flap reconstruction may be required for very large tumours with much local tissue destruction. Surgery is the treatment of choice for cases with involved regional lymph nodes when a block dissection is indicated. Overall local control rates of 95 per cent or more are to be expected after excision alone. Patients with involved resection margins should be referred for radiotherapy as these patients will be at high risk of local recurrence.

Radiotherapy

Radiotherapy is equivalent to surgery in terms of local control and is better for:

1. Tumours at sites where surgery would lead to inferior cosmesis, e.g. nasolabial fold.
2. Tumours at sites where surgery would lead to inferior functional result, e.g. lower eyelid.

Superficial X-rays or electrons are used to limit irradiation of subcutaneous tissues. Treatment can be given as a large single fraction or a course of daily treatment over 2 to 4 weeks. The former is preferred for patients who would find travelling difficult due to age or infirmity, but gives an inferior cosmetic outcome.

Chemotherapy

Topical 5-fluorouracil can cause complete regression of Bowen's disease (squamous carcinoma *in situ*) and small BCCs/SCCs, but has to be applied regularly, is inconvenient and requires careful follow-up. It is not routinely used.

Cryotherapy

Thorough and sustained freezing with liquid nitrogen is very effective for small superficial tumours. It is usually administered by a dermatologist who will have the greatest expertise.

Curettage

Suitable for small (1 cm or less), well circumscribed and superficial tumours. However, there is a higher risk of local recurrence as the margins are more likely not to be free of tumour.

Tumour-related complications

Local tissue destruction will cause loss of function, disfigurement and predispose to secondary infection and bleeding. Secondary infection will lead to discharge and discomfort and may predispose to delayed healing after surgery or radiotherapy.

Treatment-related complications

After radiotherapy an acute skin reaction is inevitable, characterized by erythema, hyperpigmentation, itching, dry desquamation and in some cases moist desquamation. This begins after 10–14 days of treatment and resolves within 2–4 weeks of completing radiotherapy.

Prognosis

It is exceptional for a patient to die from non-melanomatous skin cancer. Local control should be expected in over 95 per cent, with most recurrences being successfully salvaged by further local treatment.

Screening/prevention

The risks of ultraviolet radiation need to be appreciated, particularly by children and young adults. Avoidance of the sun during the midday period and use of sunblocks is recommended in sunny climates. Patients with a past history of skin cancer are at risk of developing others subsequently and benefit from surveillance and/or instructions regarding the early signs of a new tumour.

Melanoma

This is a rarer but more serious form of skin cancer arising from the melanocytes of the skin. It is completely curable if detected and treated at an early stage.

Epidemiology

There are 2000 new cases and 1200 deaths registered in the UK per annum and there has been a 50 per cent increase in incidence over the last decade. It is one of the few cancers that has a significant impact on young adults, 22 per cent arising in the under 40s. It is very rare in children and is twice as common in women. The geographical and racial distribution is similar to that of non-melanomatous skin cancer although melanoma does occasionally arise in dark-skinned people.

Aetiology

Ultraviolet radiation is the main causative factor, sun exposure being very important in determining risk, particularly if exposed during childhood. Additional risk factors include blond or red hair colour, and intense episodic sun exposure particularly in those who tan poorly and burn easily.

The vast majority of naevi confer no additional risk of melanoma although individuals with large numbers (> 100) are at increased risk. Dysplastic naevi may be congenital and are usually large lesions with irregular pigment and an irregular edge. Affected individuals should be watched very closely.

Pathology

The site distribution in men and women differs and is shown in Figure 19.3. Mucosal melanoma is rare and described in the upper aerodigestive tract, anus and vagina. Choroidal melanoma is also described as the pigment cells of the choroid are homologous with those of the skin. A melanoma is typically brown/black in colour due to increased melanin production by the melanocytes, frequently with irregularity of pigment at its edge or centrally (Fig. 19.4). Amelanotic tumours are seen in about 5 per

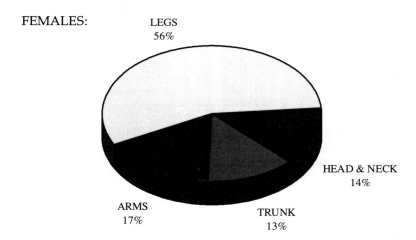

Fig. 19.3   Site distribution of malignant melanoma.

Fig. 19.4 A malignant melanoma. Note the irregular edge, uneven pigmentation and nodular component.

cent of cases. They may be nodular or flat and seen to be spreading along the superficial layers of the skin. Fifty per cent are superficial spreading melanomas and are more favourable prognostically than nodular types which have an early vertical growth phase. In advanced cases there may be associated ulceration or satellite lesions on the adjacent skin. Like hypernephromas of the kidney and neuroblastomas of the adrenal, spontaneous regression in both primary and metastatic tumours is recorded although this is seen in less than 5 per cent.

Microscopically the tumour is composed of melanocytes which invade along the superficial layers of the skin and penetrate the basement membrane into the deeper layers of the dermis. The cells characteristically stain for S100, reflecting their origin from neural crest cells. A lymphocytic infiltrate is common, reflecting a host cellular immune response.

Natural history

Melanoma may remain at a superficial spreading phase for many months before it grows into the papillary dermis, reticular dermis and sub-cutaneous fat. Nodular melanomas tend to spread into the dermis at an early stage which accounts for their poorer prognosis.

Regional lymph nodes may be involved when the melanoma invades the deeper layers of the skin.

Melanoma is a tumour which has an ability to spread to any tissue in the body. Lung and brain metastases are the most common and it is one of the few extra-abdominal tumours to spread to the bowel and its mesentery. Choroidal melanoma has a propensity to spread to the liver.

Symptoms

Presentation is usually with a pigmented skin lesion. Changes in a preceding naevus or appearance of a new pigmented lesion frequently go unnoticed, particularly if on the back, but itchiness or bleeding are particularly sinister symptoms.

Signs

The lesion will usually be on a sun-exposed area. The degree and pattern of pigmentation is variable but is characteristically irregular particularly at the edge of the lesion, and is ideally assessed with a magnifying glass. Ulceration is an ominous sign. Regional lymph nodes should be palpated for enlargement which may be due either to tumour infiltration or in reaction to the tumour/secondary infection. There may be signs of distant metastases such as hepatomegaly, pleural effusion/collapse/consolidation, or focal neurological signs. Patients with a heavy burden of metastases may have a slate grey complexion due to increased circulating melanin released by the tumour cells.

Differential diagnosis

A number of benign pigmented skin lesions may be confused with melanoma including benign naevi, seborrhoeic warts, dermatofibromata and pigmented BCC/SCC. Lentigo maligna (Hutchinson's melanotic freckle) deserves special mention. It typically occurs in the elderly on the face as a large, slow growing, superficial, pigmented and irregular lesion which represents a melanoma *in situ* and may become invasive.

Investigations
Excision biopsy

This is preferable to incision biopsy as it will provide a large specimen for detailed histological analysis and remove the lesion *in toto*, and is mandatory for any atypical pigmented lesion. Only a small macroscopic margin of normal skin is taken.

Fine needle aspiration of any enlarged regional lymph nodes

This should differentiate between reactive and metastatic enlargement.

Exclusion of metastatic disease

A chest X-ray is performed in all cases to exclude lung metastases.
   A CT scan of chest, liver and regional lymph nodes is indicated in those at high risk of metastatic disease, e.g. deeply invasive tumours.

Staging

Clark's levels measure the depth in relation to histological landmarks:

Level I   – Confined to the lamina propria.
Level II   – Reaches the papillary dermis.
Level III – Reaches the papillary/reticular dermis.

Level IV – Reaches the reticular dermis.
Level V – Reaches subcutaneous fat.

The Breslow thickness measures absolute depth in millimetres and is the distance of the deepest malignant cell from the stratum granulosum.

Treatment

Surgery

This is usually curative for localized lesions, a wide excision down to subcutaneous fat being necessary including a margin of macroscopically normal skin the size of which is dependent on the depth (if known). A centimetre of clearance for every millimetre of depth (clinical estimate or from result of previous excisional biopsy) up to a maximum of 3 cm is adequate and an immediate re-excision is necessary if the margins are not clear microscopically. A skin graft may be needed to close the defect if too large to heal by itself. In the case of subungual melanoma amputation of the digit is performed.

The role of elective regional lymph node dissection is controversial. It is not indicated for lesions 0.75 mm deep or less as the pick-up rate is very low. For lesions 3 mm or greater in depth, distant metastases are common and most will die from these rather than occult lymph node disease. There is only a limited role in intermediate depth melanomas, where lymph node dissection may improve prognosis in the small group with micrometastatic disease confined to the nodes. All patients relapsing in the regional nodes after successful local treatment and with no evidence of distant metastases should have a lymph node dissection.

Occasionally a patient will present with metastatic disease and a large fungating primary and in these circumstances local excision of the primary may be justified.

Radiotherapy

Melanomas are considered relatively radioresistant tumors. The treatment technique is the same as for other skin tumours, and there is evidence that a few large doses are more effective than a prolonged course. In the rare case of choroidal melanoma, very high doses of radiation administered using radioactive plaques sewn to the eye are curative in a high proportion. Otherwise, radiotherapy has little role as a curative treatment, being used when the patient refuses surgery or the tumour is inoperable, e.g. some mucosal melanomas. Low doses of radiation are valuable in palliating pain from skeletal metastases and focal, symptomatic metastases elsewhere.

Chemotherapy

Melanoma is not a chemosensitive tumour and is therefore incurable once distant metastasis has occurred. Adjuvant chemotherapy for high risk patients does not have any proven benefit.

The most active agents for metastatic disease are cisplatin, DTIC and vindesine. The first two are extremely unpleasant for the patient in terms of emesis and other systemic symptoms, but their use may be justified for the treatment of severe symptoms from visceral metastases which have not responded to conventional treatments. Objective responses of 30 per cent or less are to be expected.

Hormone therapy

There are reports of up to 15 per cent objective responses to the antioestrogen tamoxifen when given for metastatic disease.

Biological therapy

The recognition of spontaneous regression in melanoma and rich lymphocytic infiltrate seen in and around the lesions suggests that host immunity may play a role in the rate of growth of these tumours. Lymphokines are chemical messengers produced by T lymphocytes which stimulate lymphocyte proliferation and in turn the body's capacity for immunosurveillance. α interferon is one such lymphokine which is given subcutaneously at a dose of 3 megaunits 3–5 times weekly leading to objective responses of about 20 per cent. Similar responses have been observed to the lymphokine interleukin 2 (IL2). Both drugs are expensive and have toxicity which may prove worse than the symptoms they are being used to palliate (see below).

Tumour-related complications

Secondary infection is an uncommon complication, predisposing to local discomfort, discharge and bleeding.

Treatment-related complications

Interferon and IL2 invariably have substantial systemic toxicity. The symptoms resemble influenza and include headache, malaise, fever, rigors, myalgia, lethargy, muscular weakness, depression, confusion, hypotension, renal failure and hypothyroidism.

Prognosis

Poor prognostic factors correlate with the risk of developing distant metastases and include:

1. Deep Clark's level.
2. Large Breslow thickness (5 year survivals for lesions < 1.5 mm., 1.5–3.5 mm and > 3.5 mm are approximately 90 per cent, 70 per cent and 40 per cent respectively).
3. Ulceration.
4. Mucosal melanoma v. cutaneous (detected earlier).
5. Nodular melanoma v. superficial spreading (longer horizontal growth phase).

6. Male sex.
7. Age over 50 years.

Statistical analysis shows only the first three to be independent risk factors. Overall 5 year survival is 50–60 per cent for men, 70–80 per cent for women. The better prognosis in women is probably due to earlier detection.

Screening/prevention

Health education is again vital to inform people that episodic exposure to intense sunlight is a risk to children and young adults. People should be encouraged to visit their general practitioner for an opinion if a pigmented lesion:

1. Increases in size.
2. Changes shape or colour, particularly if pigmentation becomes irregular.
3. Develops an element of inflammation.
4. Bleeds or crusts.
5. Itches.

Regular photographs of dysplastic naevi will aid early diagnosis of malignant change and screening of other family members should be undertaken if familial.

Rare tumours

Mycosis fungoides

This is a cutaneous T-cell lymphoma with a peak incidence of 30–50 years. The eruption has a predilection for body creases, buttocks and face and is initially non-specific resembling chronic eczema or psoriasis. This stage may last for several years before progression to plaques which are well demarcated, erythematous, sometimes itchy lesions. The plaque stage progresses to the tumour stage consisting of erythematous nodules arising in the plaques or in normal skin. Erythroderma is described when the whole skin is affected, and Sezary syndrome when abnormal lymphocytes are seen in the peripheral blood (see Chapter 16). Visceral involvement is common and therefore full staging investigations are indicated. Treatment options include phototherapy with ultraviolet light, steroids, radiotherapy either locally or to the whole skin, topical or systemic chemotherapy, retinoids and interferon. The clinical course is protracted and many will die of unrelated causes.

Kaposi's sarcoma

This arises from vascular endothelial cells (see Chapter 20 for a detailed description).

Merkel cell carcinoma

The mean age at diagnosis is 65–70 years and it presents as a solitary lesion, most frequent on head and neck in sun-damaged skin. It arises from neuroendocrine cells and is locally aggressive spreading to regional lymph nodes and to distant sites. Even with combined wide local excision and post-operative radiotherapy over one-third will recur locally and about half will eventually die from their disease.

Hidradenocarcinoma

This is a carcinoma arising from the sweat glands.

Sarcoma

These arise from the soft tissues of the skin and include leiomyosarcoma, liposarcoma, malignant fibrous histiocytoma, and angiosarcoma.

Future prospects

The role of biological agents needs to be defined, either alone or combined with chemotherapy. An effective systemic adjuvant therapy capable of eradicating micrometastases is required and advances in antibody targeting of therapy may make this possible.

20

AIDS-related cancer

The acquired immune deficiency syndrome (AIDS) is a recently recognized disease which is dramatically increasing in incidence. From the oncologist's point of view, it is an important disease as about 40 per cent of sufferers can be expected to develop some form of malignant disease, which has major implications for the planning of cancer services for the future. The types of tumours encountered are particularly rare in the rest of the population and present at a relatively advanced stage in patients who do not tolerate treatment well.

Malignant disease may also be the first manifestation of infection with the human immunodeficiency virus (HIV), and should be considered in those presenting with Kaposi's sarcoma and primary cerebral lymphoma. In such patients, risk factors for AIDS should be sought:

1. Homosexual sexual contact.
2. Sexual contact with an infected heterosexual partner.
2. Intravenous drug abuse.
3. Blood transfusion in Africa or factor VIII treatment for haemophilia.

If appropriate, HIV positivity should be confirmed by a blood test.

Management problems

Coping with the diagnosis:

The patient has already been diagnosed as having an incurable illness with a poor prognosis which compounds any psychological difficulties in coping with the diagnosis of either condition alone.

Poor prognosis from the tumour and AIDS

The prognosis from the underlying tumour will usually be very poor due to the tumour presenting at an advanced stage and growing rapidly in an environment of a suppressed cellular immune system. The combination of HIV infection and malignancy will make the risk of opportunistic infection extremely high and indeed many will die from infection rather than their tumours.

Poor performance status

Patients with AIDS will often have a poor performance status which influences the treatment that they will tolerate, particularly as many present with advanced disease requiring chemotherapy that they are unlikely to tolerate.

Risk of infection to healthcare professionals

All healthcare workers who could potentially come into contact with bodily secretions should be aware of the patient's illness. Surgeons should double glove, consider wearing eyeshields during surgery, take care of any specimens obtained and notify the pathology laboratory of the risk of infection using appropriate labels. Radiographers should avoid routine use of skin tattoos, and take care with immobilization devices, e.g. bite blocks. Care should also be taken with needles and cannulae during and after administration of chemotherapy and when venepuncture is performed, and the laboratory notified of any blood specimens sent for analysis.

Predisposition to myelosuppression

Many patients will be taking zidovudine (AZT) as treatment for HIV which can cause pancytopenia and therefore exacerbate the myelosuppressive effect of radiotherapy, chemotherapy and biological agents. This may in turn limit the intensity of anti-cancer treatment that may be given.

Kaposi's sarcoma (KS)

This is the most common AIDS-related malignancy but occurs sporadically in Eastern Europeans, Africans and renal transplant patients on long-term immunosuppressants. It has not been reported in AIDS patients who contracted the disease through intravenous drug abuse. The aetiology is unknown. The tumour is derived from the vascular endothelial cells of the skin. There are usually multiple skin lesions, particularly on the lower limbs (Fig. 20.1). Extracutaneous disease is common, particularly in the oral cavity and gastrointestinal tract. The lesions have a characteristic purplish hue reflecting their vascular nature, appear as macules plaques or nodules, and may ulcerate or bleed. Spread may occur to the regional lymph nodes or distant sites such as liver and lungs. Biopsy to confirm the diagnosis is rarely necessary due to its typical appearance and frequency in AIDS patients. KS may lead directly to death when there is extensive gastrointestinal involvement leading to haemorrhage. Otherwise, most will die of other AID-related complications. Indications for active management of KS lesions include:

1.   Pain.
2.   Ulceration.

Fig. 20.1 Multiple plaques and nodules of Kaposi's sarcoma arising on the lower limbs of an AIDS patient (Courtesy of Dr R. Thomas).

3. Bleeding.
4. Oedema.
5. Disfigurement and stigma felt by patient.
6. Mass effects, e.g. upper airways obstruction.

KS is a radiosensitive tumour and although it is difficult to assess response due to residual pigmentation, there is usually a visible regression in terms of flattening of the lesion and relief of symptoms with 60–70 per cent attaining a complete response. A single fraction is suitable for cutaneous sites. Candida superinfection of mucosal surfaces and enhanced radiation mucositis are problems when the oral cavity is irradiated. Immunotherapy has also been used in KS due to:

1. Observed regression of KS in renal transplant patients with a decrease in their immunosuppression.
2. Anti-tumour, anti-viral effects of some biological modifiers.
3. Recognized spontaneous regression of KS (4 per cent) in the more immunocompetent patients.

Up to 40 per cent respond to high dose interferon with occasional complete responses. Objective responses have also been seen with chemotherapy. The drugs used are chosen to minimize the risk of myelosuppression and systemic toxicity. Bleomycin combined with vincristine is effective in these respects and is usually well tolerated by patients.

Primary cerebral lymphoma (see also
Chapters 12 and 16)

This is an extremely rare primary extranodal site of lymphoma in the general population but relatively more common in AIDS patients. It usually arises in the cerebral hemispheres and may be multifocal. Histologically it is a high grade B cell non-Hodgkin's lymphoma which infiltrates widely and may cross to the contralateral hemisphere. CSF dissemination down subarachnoid space will lead to nerve root deposits in the spine. It presents with focal or non-specific signs originating from the affected part of the brain. It must be distinguished from an opportunistic CNS infection such as toxoplasmosis or tuberculosis to which AIDS patients are susceptible. The diagnosis is made by craniotomy and biopsy supplemented by whole body CT scan and bone marrow trephine for staging as for lymphoma elsewhere. The tumour is not particularly sensitive to either radiotherapy or chemotherapy. The preferred treatment is whole brain irradiation, with chemotherapy for those of good performance status. Intrathecal methotrexate and ara-C may be used for proven spinal metastases. Primary cerebral lymphoma has an extremely poor prognosis in patients with AIDS.

Non-Hodgkin's lymphoma

These are usually high grade lymphomas, frequently resembling Burkitt's lymphoma, most presenting with stage 4 disease with extranodal involvement. 'B' symptoms such as fever may mask or be confused with an opportunistic infection. Treatment is with combination chemotherapy such as CHOP, but tolerance of such treatment is a problem due to bone marrow suppression and poor performance status of most patients. Despite a good initial response to treatment, this is often short-lived and the prognosis remains very poor.

Other tumours

Possible increases in incidence have also been described for:

1. Carcinoma of the tongue.
2. Carcinoma of the anus.
3. Hodgkin's disease.
4. Testicular tumours.
5. Hepatocellular carcinoma.

Many of these tumours are thought to have a viral aetiology (e.g. human papilloma virus and carcinoma of the anus, lymphoma and Epstein–Barr virus) which may account for their prevalence in this immunosuppressed population.

21

Carcinoma of unknown primary

Some patients are diagnosed as having disseminated cancer but with no evidence of the site of origin, many presenting with their disease as an incidental finding, e.g. enlarged cervical lymph node or multiple metastases on chest X-ray. Their management is a difficult problem, the oncologist having to determine whether the patient has a curable tumour such as a teratoma or lymphoma, or one that can benefit from some non-toxic systemic therapy, e.g. a hormone responsive cancer such as from the breast or prostate. After taking a history, patients should undergo a detailed physical examination including the skin, thyroid, breasts, peripheral lymph node groups (cervical chains, Waldeyer's ring, supraclavicular fossae, axillae and groins), rectum including prostate and the testes/ovaries/cervix. If the patient has presented with lymphadenopathy, the region which drains to those nodes should be examined thoroughly.

Differential diagnosis

The most likely primary sites vary with histology:

Histological type	Most likely sites of primary
Adenocarcinoma	Lung, gastrointestinal tract (stomach, colon, pancreas) breast, ovary.
Squamous carcinoma	Lung, head and neck.

Anaplastic tumours are mainly poorly differentiated carcinomas, the rest being undifferentiated teratomas, lymphoma, melanoma (particularly amelanotic variant), sarcomas and neuroendocrine tumours.

Investigations

Patients with distant metastases should not undergo exhaustive investigation in search of a primary that is in any case likely to be incurable.

Biopsy

The priority is to obtain a sizable piece of tissue from a part of the tumour that is not necrotic so that an accurate histological analysis is possible with enough tissue remaining for immunocytochemistry.

Immunocytochemistry

Some tissues have staining characteristics depending on their embryological origin and constituent cells:

α foetoprotein – teratomas, hepatomas.
β human chorionic gonadotrophin – teratomas, choriocarcinomas.
Prostate specific antigen (PSA) – carcinomas of the prostate.
CA125 – carcinomas of the ovary.
Leucocyte common antigen/Ki-1 antigen – lymphomas.
Pancytokeratin/epithelial membrane antigen – squamous carcinomas.
Desmin/myoglobin – rhabdomyosarcomas.
Neurone specific enolase – neuroblastomas, primitive neuroectodermal tumours.
Calcitonin – medullary carcinomas of the thyroid.
Thyroglobulin – follicular carcinomas of the thyroid.
S100 – melanomas, small cell lung cancers.
Cromogranin – carcinoids.

Cytogenetic studies

These are of value in tumours arising in children and adolescents as many tumours have characteristic chromosomal abnormalities, e.g. translocations in Ewing's sarcoma (t11;22), rhabdomyosarcoma (t2;13), non-Hodgkin's lymphoma (t8;14).

Radiological investigations

Chest X-ray will help to exclude a lung primary and pulmonary metastases. Bilateral mammography should be considered in women with adenocarcinoma of unknown primary to exclude an occult breast primary which would be amenable to aggressive locoregional therapy or hormone manipulation. An abdominopelvic ultrasound will allow assessment of the ovaries in women, the kidneys, the pancreas and the liver as a site of metastases. A transrectal ultrasound should be performed if the prostate feels suspicious.

Blood tests

A normal prostate specific antigen makes carcinoma of the prostate unlikely. Other useful markers include CA125 in women to exclude carcinoma of the ovary, α foetoprotein and β human chorionic gonadotrophin to exclude a germ cell tumour.

Other investigations

Patients presenting with squamous carcinoma in lymph nodes draining the head and neck region must be referred to an ENT surgeon for a nasoendoscopy as the patient may still have a curable occult primary cancer.

Management

The patient should be managed according to their age, general condition, site and stage of disease and symptomatology. In cases of widespread distant metastases, local treatment directed towards symptom relief is likely to be most appropriate as the patient will be incurable. The patient should be treated with curative intent if there are distant metastases and the tumour is particularly chemosensitive as in teratoma and lymphoma, or if there are regional lymph node metastases from a tumour which may be cured by aggressive local therapy, e.g. in the head and neck, breast. For this reason, women presenting with isolated axillary lymphadenopathy containing adenocarcinoma and no other primary site should be assumed to have an occult carcinoma of the breast and treated with tamoxifen and wide local excision of any mammographically visible tumour.

22

Oncological emergencies

There are few conditions in the management of malignant disease which are true emergencies. However, it is important to identify those patients in whom urgent treatment is required. The following conditions can be associated with rapid deterioration and even death, and should be considered emergency situations.

- Hypercalcaemia.
- Spinal cord or cauda equina compression.
- Superior vena cava obstruction.
- Neutropenic sepsis.
- Tumour lysis syndrome.

Hypercalcaemia

Malignant hypercalcaemia is the most common cause of a raised serum calcium in practice. It is associated in particular with lung cancer, breast cancer, prostatic cancer and myeloma. It is generally found in patients with disseminated metastatic disease although this is not essential.

Aetiology

There is increasing evidence that hypercalcaemia associated with malignancy is due principally to the effects of chemical agents released by the tumour which disturb the normal mechanisms of calcium balance. A number of chemicals have been identified but no single agent has yet seen defined. The effect of these substances is to have actions similar to parathyroid hormone and they include parathormone-like peptides, prostaglandins, interleukins and tumour growth factor (TGF)β. The result is osteoclast activation and mobilization of calcium from bones.

Symptoms

These include anorexia, nausea, vomiting, constipation, confusion, polyuria, thirst, polydipsia and bone pains.

Signs

There are usually no specific physical signs. The patient may appear drowsy and have signs of confusion and if established can become considerably dehydrated.

Differential diagnosis

Other causes of a similar constellation of symptoms may include diabetes mellitus causing polyuria, polydipsia and confusion, cerebral metastases, hepatic or renal failure or neutropenic sepsis.

Investigations

The diagnosis is made on the basis of a raised serum calcium. It is important to correct the total level for the serum albumin which is often low in patients with advanced malignant disease. The simple correction is to add to the serum calcium level in mmol/l 0.02 for every g/l of albumin below 40 which is the conventional standardization level. For example, a reading of calcium at 2.3 mmol/l with an albumin of 30 gives a corrected serum albumin of 2.5 mmol/l. The usual range is between 2.1 and 2.6 mmol/l.

Treatment

There are two components to the treatment of malignant hypercalcaemia:

1. Correction of dehydration and establishing good urine flow. An intravenous infusion of normal saline giving 1 litre every 6 hours should be established. Careful attention to fluid balance is essential particularly in the elderly who may easily become fluid overloaded. Frusemide may be added which, in addition to acting as a diuretic, also promotes urinary excretion of calcium. Thiazides should be avoided as they increase calcium reabsorption.
2. Specific therapy to reduce calcium levels. The management of hypercalcaemia in these patients has been revolutionized in recent years by the introduction of the diphosphonates which are a class of drugs acting primarily through stabilization of osteoclast activity. They are given by short intravenous infusion once good urine flow has been established. The two drugs currently available are APD and clodronate.

With the advent of diphosphonates the use of other drugs in this condition such as calcitonin, mithramycin or steroids has become of historical interest only.

Unfortunately although rapid correction of serum calcium is often possible with the above approach rebound hypercalcaemia is also very common and regular diphosphonate infusions may be required.

The ultimate prognosis for malignant hypercalcaemia is poor with most patients who present with this surviving for only a few months, succumbing to either refractory hypercalcaemia or the effects of wide-spread malignancy.

Spinal cord and cauda equina compression

This condition arises most commonly as a result of extradural tumour, typically secondary to carcinoma of the lung, breast or prostate. It should be treated as an emergency because the outcome in terms of final neurological disability is determined by the speed of diagnosis and treatment.

Aetiology

Extradural metastases are usually a result of blood-borne dissemination. Less often paravertebral tumour or tumour within the vertebral body may infiltrate directly into the spinal canal.

Symptoms

Spinal cord compression presents with neurological symptoms of weakness and reduced or altered sensation below the site of cord damage. This is accompanied by constipation and hesitancy in micturition leading to urinary retention.

Cauda equina compression similarly presents with weakness and sphincter disturbance. The sensory disturbance may be of reduced or altered sensation but also nerve root pain affecting the lumbosacral segments.

Signs

Spinal cord compression causes a spastic paraparesis, or if affecting the cervical spine quadriparesis, with a cut-off of sensory changes corresponding to the anatomical level of the compression – a sensory level. In contrast cauda equina compression will result in a flaccid paraparesis with loss of sensation in a dermatome pattern affecting the lumbosacral segments (the lower limbs and buttocks). Reflexes are increased with cord compression and plantars extensor while with cauda equina compression reflexes are reduced or lost with flexor plantar responses.

Sphincter function may be disturbed and with cauda equina compression a distended bladder may be palpable and anal tone will be lax.

Differential diagnosis

This will include intrinsic spinal cord tumours and paraneoplastic neuropathies.

Transverse myelitis will give a similar clinical picture to cord compression and in cancer patients may be due to viral infection and rarely as a side effect of chemotherapy or radiotherapy.

Other unrelated causes include prolapsed intervertebral disc, subacute combined degeneration of the cord and a parasagittal intracranial tumour.

Investigations

Urgent investigations are required to confirm the diagnosis. Plain X-rays of the spine may demonstrate associated vertebral disease. The definitive investigation is either a myelogram combined with CT scanning at the level of obstruction, as shown in Figure 22.1, or MRI of the spine. The latter where available is preferable being less invasive for the patient and giving more information of the precise extent of spinal canal involvement.

Treatment

In the presence of a known histologically confirmed malignancy treatment should proceed immediately with the following:

1. All patients should start on high dose steroids using dexamethasone 4 mg qds with, if necessary, prophylactic cimetidine or misoprostol and monitoring of urine for diabetes in those with borderline glucose tolerance.
2. Definitive treatment will usually be local radiotherapy starting on the same day as the diagnosis is made. A course of 20–30 Gy over 1 to 2 weeks will usually be prescribed.
3. Certain patients should be referred for surgery. These are those where

(a)   **(b)**

Fig. 22.1 Spinal cord compression demonstrated by (a) myelogram and (b) CT scan. Note the greater detail obtained with the CT which shows tumour destruction of the vertebral body and spread outside the vertebra.

there is instability of the spinal column with extensive vertebral collapse or spondilolisthesis.

4. Certain patients may be more appropriately treated with chemotherapy, in particular those with lymphoma, small cell lung cancer and germ cell tumours who have not been previously treated.
5. In addition appropriate general measures should continue. Patients with sphincter disturbance may require catheterization and analgesia should be given as necessary.
6. Active physiotherapy and rehabilitation is a further important component of the management to optimize the chances of neurological recovery.

When cord or cauda equina compression is the presenting feature of a malignant condition it is important to establish a histological diagnosis. This can usually be achieved by a needle biopsy of the affected region performed under CT control.

Prognosis

Survival following cord compression is principally defined by the underlying condition but since it is often a reflection of disseminated disease it is usually measured in only a few months from diagnosis.

The prognosis for neurological recovery is dependent almost entirely on the speed of diagnosis and instigation of treatment. In patients who are mobile at the start of treatment the majority (85 per cent) will walk after treatment. In contrast less than 15 per cent of paraplegic patients will regain useful neurological function despite intensive treatment. For this reason there should be a high index of suspicion for this condition, particularly in patients known to have metastatic disease with urgent referral to a specialist centre for treatment.

Superior vena cava obstruction

This refers to a clinical picture arising from a large mediastinal tumour mass causing obstruction to venous return to the right side of the heart and is often associated with other symptoms of mediastinal compression including dysphagia and stridor.

Aetiology

Any tumour involving the mediastinum may be the cause. The most common cause is carcinoma of the bronchus. In young patients in particular it is important to consider malignant lymphomas and germ cell tumours. Rarely a thymic tumour or retrosternal thyroid tumour may be the cause.

Post-mortem studies suggest that in most patients although mechanical obstruction to venous flow may be the first event thrombosis within the large veins inevitably follows although emboli are almost unknown.

Symptoms

Dyspnoea, stridor or dysphagia may be presenting symptoms. Intracranial venous congestion may cause headache or confusion. There may be swelling of the face, neck and arms.

Signs

Oedema of the face, neck and arms may be apparent with fixed engorged jugular veins and dilatation of superficial skin veins over the chest, neck, face and upper limbs. Typical appearances are shown in Figure 22.2. There may be obvious respiratory distress or stridor. A tumour mass may be palpable arising out of the mediastinum in the supraclavicular fossae. Papilloedema may be present on fundoscopy.

Investigations

A chest X-ray will usually demonstrate a mediastinal mass which will be better defined on CT scanning. Unless a diagnosis of malignancy has already been made it is important to obtain a tissue diagnosis if at all possible. Other readily accessible disease sites should be sought such as a peripheral lymph node. If the mediastinum is the only site of disease then a needle biopsy under CT control will usually be possible. More invasive approaches are usually avoided because of the theoretical risk of excessive haemorrhage from the area of raised venous pressure.

Fig. 22.2   Features of superior vena cava obstruction with arm and facial oedema, distended veins, plethora and conjunctival suffusion.

Treatment

Immediate treatment should take the form of high dose steroids using dexamethasone 4 mg qds.

Definitive treatment will be either radiotherapy or chemotherapy. Where a diagnosis of lymphoma or germ cell tumour is made further staging investigations should be completed as soon as possible followed by immediate chemotherapy. In small cell lung cancer chemotherapy may also be the treatment of choice unless there has been previous exposure to chemotherapy or the patient is elderly or frail. All other patients should receive a course of radiotherapy to the mediastinum.

Prognosis

The prognosis of superior vena cava obstruction depends on the underlying condition and in itself this is not a poor prognostic factor. For this reason it is important to identify those patients with lymphoma and germ cell tumour so that correct radical treatment can be given despite the acute nature of their presentation.

Most patients will benefit symptomatically from local treatment although recurrence of symptoms may occur at a later date.

Neutropenic sepsis

Neutropenic sepsis is a major hazard and the principal cause of treatment-related death associated with the use of cancer chemotherapy. However, if promptly identified and aggressively treated most episodes can be successfully controlled.

Aetiology

Neutropenia will occur after most chemotherapy treatment and may also be a problem with irradiation of large areas of the spine. Bone marrow infiltration by tumour is a further cause. Life-threatening infection is most likely to occur when the total neutrophil count falls below 1.0 x 10^9/l. The major cause of infection is from host organisms in the bowel or skin. The presence of a central venous line is a further risk factor. The common pathogens are gram negative bacteria such as *E. coli, Klebsiella* and *Pseudomonas* and gram positive organisms including *Staphylococcus aureus, Staphylococcus epidermidis* and *Streptococcus faecalis.* Less often the organism may be an anaerobe, pneumocystis carinii, cytomegalovirus or candidiasis.

Symptoms

The patient may be initially asymptomatic or have non-specific symptoms such as malaise and anorexia. Specific symptoms related to a site of infection may include dysuria, cough or sore throat.

Signs

Any fever over 38° in a patient with less than $1.0 \times 10^9/l$ neutrophils should be treated as due to systemic infection. There may be specific signs of infection in the oropharynx or chest. Sites of intravenous catheters should be carefully inspected for erythema or discharge. In more severe cases there may be obvious septicaemic shock with hypotension and tachycardia.

Investigations

Any patient who is at risk of neutropenia and found to be febrile requires an urgent blood count. If a low white count is confirmed blood cultures, a midstream urine, throat swab and chest X-ray are required together with swabs from other clinically relevent sites such as a catheter or cannula site and collection of sputum if produced.

Treatment

Intravenous antibiotics should be instigated as a matter of urgency. The results of cultures should not be awaited as life-threatening septicaemia may develop if there is any delay. The precise antibiotic combination to be used will be guided by individual hospital antibiotic policies but will take the form of broad spectrum cover against both gram negative and positive organisms. Typical combinations are an aminoglycoside with an extended spectrum penicillin, e.g. gentamicin or amikacin and carbenicillin, ticarcillin or piperacillin. Alternatively a single agent cephalosporin may be used such as ceftazidime or cefotaxime. If the fever does not settle after 48 hours and there have been no positive results from culture then it may be necessary to add metronidazole for anaerobic organisms or amphotericin for fungi. If there is clinical evidence for pneumocystis then treatment with high dose cotrimoxazole will be required.

Once the results of cultures become available then antibiotics can be adjusted appropriately. They should be continued for at least 5 days or for 48 hours after the fever has settled, whichever is the longer period.

In patients at high risk of infection then antibiotic prophylaxis is recommended. This includes those with leukaemia and lymphoma undergoing intensive chemotherapy. Daily cotrimoxazole is as good as more complex regimes together with oral antifungal agents such as nystatin or amphotericin.

Tumour lysis syndrome

This is a syndrome arising as a result of rapid breakdown of large numbers of cells usually at instigation of chemotherapy for a highly sensitive tumour such as lymphoma or leukaemia. This results in extensive metabolic disturbance characterised by hyperkalaemia, hyperuricaemia, hyperphosphataemia and hypocalcaemia.

If clinically significant the syndrome may present as acute renal failure or acute cardiac arrhythmias with the risk of sudden death.

Treatment

Tumour lysis should be anticipated in any patient with a bulky lymphoma or leukaemia about to undergo chemotherapy. Preventive measures should be instigated prior to chemotherapy with 24 hours of prehydration ensuring good renal output and urine flow, and oral allopurinol should be started to prevent hyperuricaemia.

In patients who develop metabolic disturbances after chemotherapy then intravenous hydration should be continued. Alkalinization of urine with sodium bicarbonate may increase tubular excretion of potassium and phosphate. Specific measures to reduce very high levels of potassium may be required using insulin and glucose in order to prevent cardiac arrhythmias. In the most severe cases, particularly where renal function deteriorates, then dialysis may be required.

Prognosis

In most cases the metabolic sequelae of tumour lysis should be predictable and preventable. Where metabolic disturbance does occur prompt treatment is usually successful and the effects are usually self-limiting with resolution within 5–7 days of chemotherapy.

23

Palliative care

Medical care of a cancer patient does not stop when there is no curative treatment to offer and indeed over 50 per cent of 'cancer treatments' are palliative. In this area lie many of the greatest challenges of patient care – controlling pain, dyspnoea, vomiting, haemorrhage and other tumour-related symptoms.

Pain control

The incidence of pain in patients with advanced cancer is between 70 and 80 per cent. This can be effectively controlled in almost all cases by the application of simple rules governing the use of analgesics and related drugs.

1. Make a precise diagnosis of the cause of pain, e.g. whether a bone metastasis or nerve root pain.
2. Remember that many patients will have more than one pain and that pre-existing causes of pain such as arthritis will still be important.
3. Prescribe analgesics regularly, *not* as required, to prevent pain rather than wait for pain to return before the next dose.
4. Use and be familiar with a small number of drugs based on the analgesic ladder shown in Figure 23.1.
5. Consider specific cancer treatments, e.g. radiotherapy for bone pain whenever appropriate.
6. Continually reassess the response to treatment and be prepared to modify regimes as the patient's condition evolves.

The use of analgesics in this situation should be based on a simple three-step analgesic ladder progressively escalating the potency of drug used (Fig. 23.1).

Morphine

Morphine should be used when the pain is no longer responsive to a moderate strength analgesic such as regular coproxamol or codeine. The following principles apply to the use of morphine in this setting:

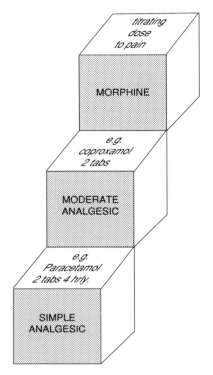

Fig. 23.1 Analgesic ladder.

1. Start treatment with regular 4 hourly morphine solution or tablets. These are much more flexible for dose titration than controlled release tablets.
2. Start with morphine a regular laxative such as codanthramer.
3. Start or be prepared to introduce a regular antiemetic such as haloperidol.
4. Slowly increase the dose from an initial 10 mg 4 hourly until pain control is achieved. Initially the dose may be doubled every 24–48 hours; beyond 60 mg 4 hourly increments of 50 per cent may be better tolerated.
5. Warn the patient that during the introduction and dose titration they may feel drowsy and that this will improve once on a stable dose.
6. Reassure the patient that addiction does not occur in this setting.

Injection

Injection of opioid drugs such as morphine does not make them more potent when equivalent doses are given and should only be considered when oral or rectal administration is not possible. Remember, however, that because of its greater bioavailability, when injected the oral dose should be approximately halved to give an equivalent analgesic action.

Controlled release morphine

Morphine tablets giving a 12 hourly release of morphine are generally preferred by patients once their dose requirements have been defined. Conversion from one morphine preparation to the other is simple as they are equivalent and a 12 hourly dose may therefore be given as a single controlled release tablet or divided into three doses of immediate release morphine at 4 hourly intervals.

If pain recurs then the cause should be investigated. Immediate release morphine may be given in addition to controlled release tablets to redefine morphine requirements or the patient changed back to 4 hourly morphine.

Spinal opioids

Epidural or intrathecal administration usually using diamorphine, may have a place in patients with very high morphine requirements or who are resistant to oral medication.

Alternatives to morphine

There are very few drugs which have advantages over morphine in this setting.

Diamorphine (diacetylmorphine)

This is preferred for injections because of its greater solubility. Otherwise it has no advantages and is converted to morphine rapidly on passing through the liver.

Phenazocine

Sometimes tolerated better in patients who are having specific side effects with morphine. It is a less flexible preparation being available in only 5 mg tablets each of which is equivalent to around 25 mg of morphine when given in a regular schedule.

Buprenorphine

May be effective in patients requiring low doses (i.e. 10 mg 4 hourly) of morphine but beyond this no greater effect of increasing doses is seen and patients will need to be switched to morphine. Its use is therefore rather limited.

Morphine-resistant pain

While the above approach will work well for most patients there is undoubtedly a group of patients whose pain is not sensitive to morphine or other opioid drugs. It is important to recognize these patients and not submit them to ever-increasing doses of morphine for no benefit. In particular musculoskeletal pains and neurogenic pains may fall into this category.

Therefore, in patients who after dose titration to 40 or 60 mg morphine 4 hourly are reporting no pain reduction with medication it is important to reconsider the further use of morphine and explore alternative approaches with coanalgesics, non-drug teatments or specific treatment such as local radiotherapy.

Coanalgesics

Coanalgesics are drugs which do not have intrinsic analgesic activity but in specific situations will help in pain relief. Examples include the following:

Non-steroidal anti-inflammatory drugs (NSAID)

Useful in bone pain and soft tissue infiltration by tumour. These include drugs such as aspirin, ibuprofen or naproxen.

Steroids

Of value in nerve root pain, raised intracranial pressure, hepatomegaly and soft tissue infiltration. Dexamethasone may be more convenient than prednisolone but both are effective in moderate doses, e.g. dexamethasone 4 mg twice daily or prednisolone 20–40 mg daily. There may be the added advantage of increased well-being experienced by many patients on taking steroids.

Anxiolytic drugs

Small doses of drugs such as diazepam may be required where anxiety is either a major component of pain or a debilitating condition in its own right.

Antidepressants

These may be required for some patients who are significantly depressed and may also be of value for neurogenic pain.

Muscle relaxants

Baclofen may be of value for muscle spasm.

Anticonvulsants

Drugs such as carbamazepine, sodium valproate or clonazepam are helpful for neurogenic pain.

Specific cancer treatments for pain control

For local pain from a growing and infiltrating tumour specific therapy aimed at a reduction in tumour bulk and growth arrest is often the most effective approach.

Radiotherapy

The treatment of choice for metastatic bone pain with over 80 per cent of patients responding to a single dose of radiation.

It is also highly effective in relieving headache due to raised intracranial pressure from primary or metastatic intracranial tumours.

In other situations where tumour is invading nerve roots or plexuses, as with an apical lung tumour invading the brachial plexus or presacral rectal tumour invading the lumbosacral plexus, radiotherapy is indicated for pain control.

Chemotherapy

This is often not as effective as irradiation for bone pain relief but in other circumstances with a chemosensitive tumour invading normal tissue it will be equally effective.

Other pain treatments

Pain may have many components to it and in particular the pain associated with malignant disease is recognized to have a major affective (emotional) component. Alternative non-drug treatments may be very successful in selected patients who do not respond well to the above approach. These may include:

- Transcutaneous electrical nerve stimulation (TENS) may be particularly valuable for neurogenic pains.
- Specific nerve blocks can be dramatically successful in selected cases.
- Neurosurgical procedures such as cordotomy, rhizotomy or thalotomy may occasionally be indicated.
- Massage including the use of heat and cold to painful and tender areas.
- Acupuncture which may be particularly successful for difficult neurogenic pains.
- Relaxation and techniques such as aromatherapy may also have a place in alleviating distress related to advanced malignancy.

Other symptoms

Because of the systemic nature of metastatic cancer many other symptoms may affect the patient with advanced cancer. These include anorexia, nausea and vomiting, constipation, sore mouth, confusion, cough and dyspnoea.

The basic principle of making a diagnosis of the precise cause for each symptom should be adhered to in order to choose the most effective treatment.

Anorexia

This may be due to anxiety, nausea, pain, liver metastases, sore mouth or uraemia, each of which may require specific treatment.

In addition appetite may be stimulated by the use of low doses of steroids such as dexamethasone 4 mg daily or prednisolone 10–20 mg daily. Progestogens such as medroxyprogesterone or megestrol may also be of value.

Nausea and vomiting

This may be a side effect of many drugs used in this situation, in particular morphine. Other potential causes include mechanical bowel obstruction, hepatic metastases, uraemia or hypercalcaemia.

In addition to correction where possible of biochemical disturbance antiemetic drugs will be required. It is important to consider a rational choice of the many drugs available based on their site of action, as shown in Table 23.1.

Table 23.1   Anti-emetic drugs in advanced cancer

Site of action	Drugs	Indication
Vomiting centre	Cyclizine	May be useful in all causes as this is the final common pathway for vomiting reflex
Chemoreceptor trigger zone	Prochlorperazine Chlorpromazine Haloperidol Metoclopramide Ondansetron	Drug induced, Metabolic, e.g. uraemia, hypercalcaemia Hepatic metastases
Peripheral	Metoclopramide Ondansetron	Gastric stasis

Constipation

This may be a side effect of drugs, in particular morphine, or related to dehydration, hypercalcaemia or mechanical restriction of the bowel from intra-abdominal or pelvic tumour.

Laxatives should be given regularly, again recognizing their different modes of action for different indications. Codanthramer which has a combination of a bowel stimulant and faecal softener is often of value.

Sore mouth

This may be due to dryness of the oral cavity as a side effect of drugs including morphine and phenothiazine antiemetics, radiotherapy to the mouth, or mucositis related to chemotherapy or candidiasis.

Oropharyngeal candidiasis can cause severe symptoms in these patients and should be treated actively with topical nystatin or amphotericin using systemic ketoconazole for resistant cases. Regular mouthwashes, sucking ice cubes, carbonated drinks or ascorbic acid are also recommended.

Confusion

This can be one of the most difficult symptoms to deal with. There is usually an identifiable cause including drugs, in particular morphine, hepatic or renal dysfunction, hypercalcaemia, hypoxia, infection or cerebral metastases.

In addition to specific attention to the above, mild sedation with low doses of a benzodiazepine may be of value. In severe cases with hallucinations then haloperidol may be required in the acute phase. However, drugs should not take the place of sympathetic psychological support and reasssurance counteracting the cycle of misinterpretation and over-reaction which builds up.

Cough and dyspnoea

This will usually arise as a result of intrathoracic tumour causing bronchial irritation or obstruction, lung collapse, lung metastases or pleural effusion. Chest infections are also common in this group of patients.

Treatment may include aspiration of effusion and antibiotics. Specific cough sedatives based on codeine linctus may be tried but are often unsuccessful as are bronchodilators unless there is preceding obstructive airways disease. Small doses of morphine (10–20 mg 4 hourly) are often the most useful and steroids may be of value in diffuse lung infiltration of lymphangitis carcinomatosa.

Common patterns are seen to emerge when considering the above symptoms. In particular many symptoms may be attributable to bio-chemical disturbance and simple investigations including blood urea and electrolytes, liver function tests and serum calcium are often rewarding in providing a cause for specific problems.

The dying patient

Inevitably there will come a time when death is imminent. This may require changes in medication to minimize the physical distress for both the patient and their relatives. The following points should be considered:

1. Diminishing levels of consciousness will require a switch from oral medication. It is rarely necessary to give drugs intravenously or intramuscularly and the subcutaneous route should be chosen. If the patient is expected to succumb within a day or so intermittent injections may be acceptable but it is often easier and less traumatic to set up a continuous infusion pump. Diamorphine or morphine can be given by this route (remembering to reduce the oral dose by 50 per cent) and if anti-emetics are required haloperidol or metoclopramide can be added to the infusion. Alternatively these may be given in suppository form.

2. There may be terminal agitation and restlessness. This is best treated by rectal diazepam or using haloperidol or midazolam in the subcutaneous infusion.

3. Pooling of secretions may make respiration unpleasantly noisy and uncomfortable. This is best controlled with subcutaneous hyoscine in doses of 0.2–0.4 mg.

4. Many patients continue to be left on large numbers of oral medications most of which are irrelevant in these final hours. It is important therefore to review carefully all medication and in general most routine oral medical treatments such as antihypertensives, anti-inflammatory drugs, laxatives and H2 antagonists can be discontinued without causing distress to the patient or hastening death.

5. Acute deaths are unusual in oncology but rarely a tumour may erode a large enough blood vessel to cause acute haemorrhage. The typical sites for this are the carotid artery in the neck, femoral artery in the groin or an intrapulmonary vessel. These are inevitably terminal events and can cause considerable distress. Sedation with parenteral diamorphine and local pressure to control blood loss should be administered. A dark-coloured blanket is also of great value in masking the dramatic loss of blood.

6. It is always distressing following a chronic illness and inevitable death for the final moments to be submitted to inappropriate resuscitation procedures. It is important therefore that clear policies regarding resuscitation are given to those caring for the patient arrived at after discussion with relatives and the patients themselves.

Bibliography

Suggested further reading

The Oxford Textbook of Palliative Medicine
Eds Doyle, D., Hanks, G.W.C. and MacDonald, N.
Oxford University Press
Oxford 1993
ISBN 0 19 262028 2

Cancer Chemotherapy: An Introduction
3rd edition
Priestman, T.J.
Springer-Verlag
Berlin 1989
ISBN 3 540 19551 3

Treatment of cancer
2nd edition
Eds Sikora, K. and Halnan, K.E.
Chapman & Hall Medical
London 1990
ISBN 0 412 29400 1

Cancer and its Management
2nd edition
Souhami, R. and Tobias, J.
Blackwell Scientific Publications
Oxford 1987
ISBN 0 632 01373 7

Clinical Oncology
Pocket Consultant series
2nd edition
Sweetenham, J.W. *et al.*
Blackwell Scientific Publications
Oxford 1989
ISBN 0 632 02449 6

The Oxford Textbook of Medicine
2nd edition
Eds Weatherall, D.J., Ledingham, J.G.G. and Warrell, D.A.
Oxford University Press
Oxford 1990
ISBN 0 19 261551 3

TNM Atlas: Illustrated Guide to the TNM/pTNM Classification of Malignant Tumours
3rd edition, 4th corrected printing
Springer-Verlag
Berlin 1993
ISBN 3 540 17721 3

Index